Instructor's Manual to Accompany

PATHOLOGY

for the Health-Related Professions   Second Edition

Ivan Damjanov, M.D., Ph.D.
Professor
Department of Pathology
University of Kansas
School of Medicine
Kansas City, Kansas

W.B. Saunders Company
A Division of Harcourt Brace & Company
Philadelphia   London   Toronto   Montreal   Sydney   Tokyo

W.B. SAUNDERS COMPANY

A Division of Harcourt Brace & Company

The Curtis Center
Independence Square West
Philadelphia, Pennsylvania 19106

INSTRUCTOR'S MANUAL TO ACCOMPANY
PATHOLOGY FOR THE HEALTH-RELATED PROFESSIONS, Second Edition   ISBN 0-7216-8119-0

Copyright © 2000, 1996 by W.B. Saunders Company

All rights reserved. No part of this publication may be reproduced or transmitted in any form or by any means electronic or mechanical including photocopy, recording or any information storage and retrieval system without permission in writing from the publisher.

Printed in the United States of America

Last digit is the print number: 9 8 7 6 5 4 3 2 1

Contents

	Preface	v
Chapter 1	Cell Pathology	1
Chapter 2	Inflammation	5
Chapter 3	Immunopathology	8
Chapter 4	Neoplasia	13
Chapter 5	Genetic and Developmental Diseases	18
Chapter 6	Fluid and Hemodynamic Disorders	22
Chapter 7	The Cardiovascular System	27
Chapter 8	The Respiratory System	31
Chapter 9	The Hematopoietic and Lymphoid System	36
Chapter 10	The Gastrointestinal System	41
Chapter 11	The Liver and Biliary Tract	46
Chapter 12	The Pancreas	52
Chapter 13	The Urinary Tract	57
Chapter 14	The Male Reproductive System	61
Chapter 15	The Female Reproductive System	66
Chapter 16	The Breast	73
Chapter 17	The Endocrine System	77
Chapter 18	The Skin	82
Chapter 19	Bones and Joints	86
Chapter 20	Muscles	90
Chapter 21	The Nervous System	95
Chapter 22	The Eye	100
Chapter 23	The Ear	103

PREFACE

This collection of more than 500 questions and some 200 clinicopathologic case studies was prepared as an instructor's manual to help teachers using the textbook *Pathology for the Health-Related Professions*. The manual follows the outline of the textbook. Accordingly, it is divided into 23 chapters, each of which contains between one and three dozen questions. Shorter textbook chapters are accompanied by fewer questions, whereas the material of longer chapters receive more attention. Nevertheless, I think that each chapter contains more than enough questions for monitoring students' progress or for final evaluation.

Questions are in the form of multiple-choice questions (A-type) in which one of the five answers is correct. In addition, several chapters include matching-type questions in which one of the five lettered items must be matched with the most appropriate numbered item. These matching questions are best used in a battery of five in which case the number of lettered items (questions) equals the number of numbered items (answers). However, each numbered item could also be used individually with the same set of five lettered items. In other words, a matching question containing 10 numbered items could be transformed into 10 individual A-type questions. Needless to say, the examiner may vary each of the foils and thus double or triple the number of questions.

I hope that instructors will find this textbook useful. I also hope that it does not contain too many mistakes, factual or typographical. For all those, please do not blame anybody but the author, who will try to correct them, hopefully with your help, in the next edition.

Please direct all your comments to me by E-mail (IDAMJANO@KUMC.EDU), by regular mail, through the publisher, or even by telephone. My secretary, Stephanie Yeager, and I are looking forward to your correspondence.

Ivan Damjanov, M.D.
University of Kansas Medical Center
Kansas City, KS 66160-7410

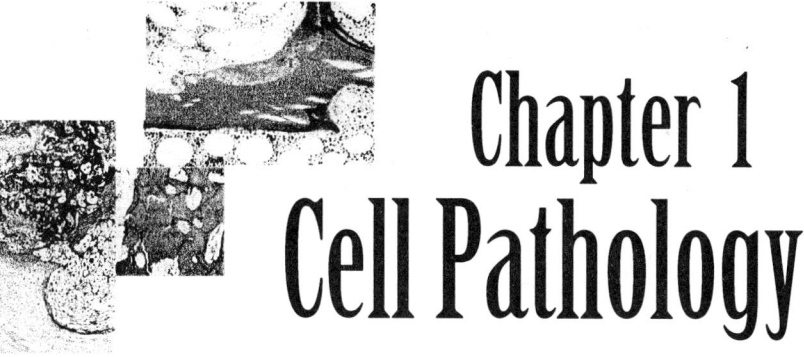

Chapter 1
Cell Pathology

Instruction: Match the numbered words or phrases with the most appropriate lettered item. Each lettered item can be used more than once.

- A. Mitochondria
- B. Lysosomes
- C. Endoplasmic reticulum
- D. Intermediate filaments
- E. Plasma membrane

1. Its rupture causes irreversible cell injury

2. Major component of the cytoskeleton

3. Precursors of heterophagosomes

4. The site of synthesis of proteins

5. Ribosomes may be attached to it

6. Major site of energy production in the cytoplasm

7. Double membranes enclosed organelles rich in oxidative enzymes

8. In epithelial cells they are composed of keratins

9. Its invaginations form endocytotic vacuoles

10. It is the site of hormone synthesis

Answers: 1. E, 2. D, 3. B, 4. C, 5. C, 6. A, 7. A, 8. D, 9. E, 10. C

Instruction: Choose the one best answer.

11. All the following are signs of irreversible cell injury except:
    - A. Apoptosis
    - B. Pyknosis
    - C. Karyorrhexis
    - D. Karyolysis
    - E. Vacuolar degeneration

    Answer: E

12. Inhibition of ATP production by hypoxia causes all the following except:
    - A. Increased production of lactic acid in the cytoplasm
    - B. Degranulation of the rough endoplasmic reticulum
    - C. Dilatation of rough endoplasmic reticulum
    - D. Swelling of the mitochondria
    - E. Alkalinization of the hyaloplasm

    Answer: E

13. Which of the following is an oxygen radical?
    - A. Hydrogen peroxide
    - B. Acid hydrolase
    - C. ATP
    - D. Carbon tetrachloride
    - E. Lipofuscin

    Answer: A

14. Which of the following organs undergoes atrophy during childhood and adolescence?
    A. Uterus
    B. Breasts
    C. Thymus
    D. Thyroid
    E. Adrenals

    Answer: C

15. Enlargement of the heart due to hypertension is a result of:
    A. Hyperplasia
    B. Hypertrophy
    C. Atrophy
    D. Metaplasia
    E. Dysplasia

    Answer: B

16. Columnar bronchial epithelium irritated by chronic exposure to cigarette smoke changes into stratified squamous epithelium. This change is an example of:
    A. Hypertrophy
    B. Hyperplasia
    C. Atrophy
    D. Metaplasia
    E. Degeneration

    Answer: D

17. Chronic hemolysis is characterized by accumulation of an iron-containing brown pigment in the cytoplasm of liver cells. This brown pigment is called:
    A. Melanin
    B. Tyrosin
    C. Hemosiderin
    D. Ceruloplasmin
    E. Bilirubin

    Answer: C

18. Which type of necrosis is found in granulomas of tuberculosis?
    A. Coagulation necrosis
    B. Liquefactive necrosis
    C. Caseous necrosis
    D. Fat necrosis
    E. Fibrinoid necrosis

    Answer: C

19. Myocardial infarct represents a form of:
    A. Dystrophic calcification
    B. Metastatic calcification
    C. Fibrinoid necrosis
    D. Coagulation necrosis
    E. Wet gangrene

    Answer: D

20. Liquefactive necrosis typically occurs following infarction of the:
    A. Heart
    B. Brain
    C. Liver
    D. Kidney
    E. Pancreas

    Answer: B

Clinicopathologic Review

Chapter 1—Cell Pathology

Symptoms/Findings	Question	Answer
A liver biopsy was performed, and the tissue was examined histologically. No chromosomes were seen in 100 liver cells.	Is this normal?	Yes. Chromosomes cannot be seen in interphase nuclei, but only during mitosis. In resting, nondividing cells, DNA and RNA are distributed in the nucleus in the form of chromatin.
The liver cells of an epileptic patient who received a daily dose of phenobarbital showed increased amounts of SER.	What is the explanation for this finding?	Phenobarbital is a drug metabolized in the SER. This organelle will undergo hyperplasia if stimulated. Increased amounts of SER in liver cells are found following chronic drug intake.
Increased amounts of SER were found by electron microscopy in testicular Leydig cells.	Is this normal?	Yes. Leydig cells synthesize sex hormones. Steroids are produced in the SER and, therefore, all steroid-producing cells normally have a well-developed SER.
Plasma cells were found to contain increased amounts of RER.	Is this normal?	Yes. Plasma cells secrete immunoglobulins which, like all other proteins for export, are synthesized on the RER.
A mercurial diuretic caused hydropic changes in the kidney cells.	How could this be explained?	Mercury is a heavy metal that inhibits enzymes in proximal kidney cells. Mercury salts, used in small amounts for therapeutic purposes, produce reversible cell injury in the form of hydropic change. In large amounts, mercury causes cell necrosis.
The pH in the liver cells of a patient was determined to be 5.2.	Is this normal?	No. Normally, the pH in liver cells is neutral to slightly alkaline (7.0–7.3). Acidification of the cytoplasm is evidence of cell injury, as in anoxia. Anoxia leads to overproduction of lactic acid through anaerobic glycolysis. This occurs after aerobic phosphorylation has been inhibited owing to lack of oxygen.

Copyright © 2000 by W.B. Saunders Company. All rights reserved.

Symptoms/Findings (con't)	Question (con't)	Answer (con't)
Myelin figures were found in liver cells exposed to carbon tetrachloride.	What is the significance of these myelin figures?	Myelin figures represent concentrically layered membranes resembling the myelin of peripheral nerves. These are structures formed from damaged cell membranes and are commonly found in injured cells. However, they are also found within lysosomes in individuals with lipid storage diseases, like Tay-Sachs disease.
A small heart in a 90-year-old woman was found to be full of lipofuscin.	What is the diagnosis?	A small heart and accumulation of lipofuscin (the so-called brown pigment of aging) are signs of senile atrophy. Similar changes may, however, be seen in debilitated and emaciated younger patients as well.
The left ventricle of the heart was 2.5 cm thick (normal 1.5 cm).	What is the significance of this finding?	This thickening of the wall of the left ventricle indicates hypertrophy. If the aortic outflow tract and the valves are normal, the myocardial hypertrophy is most likely secondary to arterial hypertension.
Large amounts of brown pigment were noted in a liver biopsy specimen obtained from a man who had hemolytic anemia.	What is the brown pigment?	The brown pigment in the liver is hemosiderin. Hemosiderin, an iron-containing pigment, is derived from hemoglobin of hemolyzed red blood cells.
A patient with myocardial infarction had no heartbeat for 5 minutes but was resuscitated. He remained unconscious and had to be maintained on a respirator.	Is this man alive?	The argument whether this man is alive or dead could be entertained forever. However, he is most likely "brain-dead." If respiratory support was discontinued, he would not be able to breathe and would die shortly thereafter.
The wall of the urinary bladder in a patient with prostatic enlargement was found to be thick and trabeculated.	What is the diagnosis of the bladder and the prostatic lesion?	The thickening of the bladder wall is secondary to smooth muscle cell hypertrophy, required to overcome the obstruction of the urinary outflow tract. The prostate is most likely enlarged owing to hormonally induced hyperplasia.

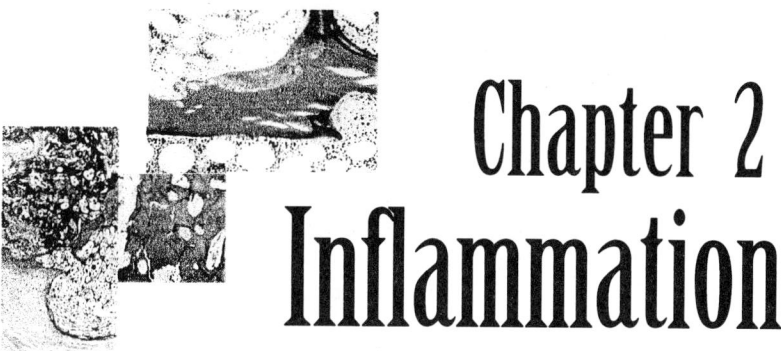

Chapter 2
Inflammation

Instruction: Match the numbered words or phrases with the most appropriate lettered item. Each lettered item can be used more than once.

    A. Polymorphonuclear leukocytes
    B. Eosinophils
    C. Basophils
    D. Macrophages
    E. Platelets

1. They have segmented nuclei, usually composed of three lobes. Because their cytoplasmic granules stain both with hematoxylin and eosin, i.e., neutrally, they are also called neutrophils.

2. These cells represent the primary defense system against bacteria.

3. These contain cytoplasmic granules that stain pink with eosin. These granules contain crystals visible by electron microscopy.

4. These cells are most prominent in allergic reactions and inflammation caused by parasitic infections.

5. The derivatives of these cells are most prominent in tissues affected by allergic reactions mediated by IgE, such as hay fever.

6. Mast cells are derivatives of these circulating blood cells.

7. These phagocytic mononuclear cells, also called histiocytes, are typical features of chronic inflammation.

8. They represent cytoplasmic fragments of megakaryocytes.

9. These cells participate in the formation of granulomas.

10. They are essential for blood clotting.

Answers: 1. A, 2. A, 3. B, 4. B, 5. C, 6. C, 7. D, 8. E, 9. D, 10. E

Instruction: Choose the one best answer.

11. All of the following are cardinal signs of inflammation except:
    A. Calor (heat)
    B. Rubor (redness)
    C. Tumor (swelling)
    D. Dolor (pain)
    E. Odor (smell)

Answer: E

12. Dilatation of arterioles results in:
    A. Anemia
    B. Hyperemia
    C. Vasoconstriction
    D. Hemorrhage
    E. Ischemia

Answer: B

13. Release of histamine at the site of inflammation causes:
    A. Increased vascular permeability
    B. Decreased vascular permeability
    C. Accumulation of neutrophils
    D. Accumulation of platelets
    E. Activation of the complement system

Answer: A

14. Which of the following blood components has fibrinolytic activity and can lyze thrombi?
    A. Bradykinin
    B. Histamine
    C. Complement membrane attack complex
    D. Plasmin
    E. Prostaglandin

    Answer: D

15. Aspirin can inhibit some aspects of inflammation by inhibiting the synthesis of:
    A. Histamine
    B. Prostaglandin and thromboxane
    C. Serotonin
    D. Hageman factor
    E. Arachidonic acid

    Answer: B

16. A bacterial throat infection ("strepthroat") is associated with a white exudate surrounded by reddened mucosa. This is an example of:
    A. Serous inflammation
    B. Fibrinous inflammation
    C. Abscess
    D. Gangrene
    E. Ulcerative inflammation

    Answer: B

17. The center of an abscess contains:
    A. Caseous necrosis
    B. Calcification
    C. Pus
    D. Eosinophils
    E. Fibrous tissue

    Answer: C

18. Granulomas consist of all the following cells except:
    A. Lymphocytes
    B. Macrophages
    C. Epithelioid cells
    D. Giant cells
    E. Polymorphonuclear leukocytes

    Answer: E

19. Which of the following is the most common cause of delayed healing of a skin wound caused by a traffic accident?
    A. lack of vitamin
    B. Lack of vitamin C
    C. Zinc deficiency
    D. Infection
    E. Diabetes mellitus

    Answer: D

20. Hypertrophic scars are called:
    A. Granuloma
    B. Granulation tissue
    C. Proud flesh
    D. Keloid
    E. Dehiscence

    Answer: D

Clinicopathologic Review

Chapter 2—Inflammation

Symptoms/Findings	Question	Answer
A slap on the face produced an area of redness on the cheek.	Why did the face become red?	This redness reflects active hyperemia that is mediated by vasodilatation (i.e., relaxation of smooth muscle cells in the arterioles and flooding of the capillary network with blood).

Symptoms/Findings *(con't)*	Question *(con't)*	Answer *(con't)*
White blood cells (WBCs) were attached to the endothelial cells of small blood vessels in the area of inflammation.	What is the reason for this pavementing?	The attachment of WBCs to the endothelial cells is a consequence of changes in blood flow that marginalize the WBCs in the blood. In addition, the attachment of WBCs to endothelial cells is mediated by activated receptors on both cell types.
The WBCs recovered from the urethral discharge of a man with gonorrhea were found to contain bacteria.	How did the bacteria enter the WBCs?	The bacteria (gonococci) were actively phagocytized by the WBCs.
When tissue involved by an allergic inflammation was examined in sections stained with hematoxylin and eosin, many eosinophils, but no basophils, were seen.	Is this what one would expect?	Yes. In tissue sections, eosinophils can be readily recognized owing to their granules, which stain pink with eosin. The granules of basophils are not evident in sections stained with hematoxylin and eosin. In order to visualize basophils, one must stain tissues with a metachromatic stain (e.g., Giemsa stain).
An inflammation lasted 2 days.	Is this an acute or chronic inflammation?	Inflammations that last a few hours or days are classified as acute.
A kidney was affected by inflammation for 2 months.	What types of cells would one expect to find in this tissue?	This is a chronic inflammation. One thus would expect to find lymphocytes, macrophages, and plasma cells. Fibroblastic scarring also could be prominent.
The pericardium was covered with a shaggy, soft, red material that could be removed easily.	Is this material fibrin or fibrous tissue?	This is most likely fibrin tinged with blood. In contrast to fibrous tissue, which is composed of collagen, fibrin is soft.
Straw-colored clear fluid was removed from the left hemithorax of a man with viral pleuritis.	What is this inflammation called?	This type of pleural effusion is typical of serous inflammation.

Chapter 3
Immunopathology

Instruction: Match the numbered words or phrases with the most appropriate lettered item. Each lettered item can be used more than once.

    A. Type I hypersensitivity reaction
    B. Type II hypersensitivity reaction
    C. Type III hypersensitivity reaction
    D. Type IV hypersensitivity reaction
    E. Graft versus host reaction

1. An important complication of bone marrow transplantation
2. Hay fever
3. Hemolytic anemia due to hypersensitivity to a drug that acts as a hapten
4. Systemic lupus erythematosus
5. Contact dermatitis to rubber gloves
6. Asthma
7. Poison ivy skin reaction
8. Polyarteritis nodosa
9. Goodpasture's syndrome
10. Graves' disease
11. Myasthenia gravis
12. Hypersensitivity to mycobacterium tuberculosis
13. Atopic dermatitis
14. Anaphylactic shock following bee sting
15. Serum sickness
16. Blood transfusion reaction
17. Rejection of skin xenograft
18. Rh incompatibility reaction in the fetus

Answers: 1. E, 2. A, 3. B, 4. C, 5. D, 6. A, 7. D, 8. C, 9. B, 10. B, 11. B, 12. D, 13. A, 14. A, 15. C, 16. B, 17. D, 18. B

Instruction: Choose the one best answer.

19. Which set of lymphocytes is decreased the most in the blood of patients with AIDS?
    A. B lymphocytes
    B. T-helper lymphocytes
    C. T-suppressor/cytotoxic lymphocytes
    D. Natural killer cells
    E. Bone marrow stem cell precursor of lymphocytes

Answer: C

20. Antibodies are produced by:
    A. B lymphocytes
    B. T-suppressor/cytotoxic lymphocytes
    C. Monocytes
    D. Plasma cells
    E. Eosinophils

Answer: D

21. All the following are lymphokines produced by macrophages or T cells except:
    A. Interleukins
    B. Immunoglobulins
    C. Interferons
    D. Tumor necrosis factor
    E. Colony-stimulating factors

    Answer: B

22. Which of the following diseases is mediated by immunoglobulin E (IgE) attached to mast cells?
    A. Hay fever (allergic rhinitis)
    B. Systemic lupus erythematosus
    C. Sarcoidosis
    D. Polyarteritis nodosa
    E. Ankylosing spondylitis

    Answer: A

23. Autoimmune disease presenting with hyperthyroidism is called:
    A. Goodpasture's syndrome
    B. Sarcoidosis
    C. DiGeorge's disease
    D. Graves' disease
    E. Myasthenia gravis

    Answer: D

24. Tissue transplantation between genetically identical twins is called:
    A. Allograft
    B. Isograft
    C. Homograft
    D. Xenograft
    E. Heterograft

    Answer: B

25. All the following organs have been successfully transplanted in humans except:
    A. Brain
    B. Heart
    C. Pancreas
    D. Lungs
    E. Kidneys

    Answer: A

26. All the following are considered to be autoimmune diseases except:
    A. Systemic lupus erythematosus
    B. Multiple sclerosis
    C. Primary biliary cirrhosis
    D. Pemphigus vulgaris
    E. AIDS

    Answer: E

27. Antinuclear antibodies (ANAs) are found typically in:
    A. Systemic lupus erythematosus
    B. AIDS
    C. Graft versus host reaction
    D. Sarcoidosis
    E. Isolated deficiency of IgA

    Answer: A

28. For the diagnosis of AIDS it is important to test the patient for antibodies to:
    A. Human papillomavirus (HPV)
    B. Epstein-Barr virus (EBV)
    C. Human immunodeficiency virus (HIV)
    D. Pneumocystis carinii
    E. Mycobacterium avium intracellulare

    Answer: C

29. Which of the following is a common feature of AIDS?
    A. Burkitt's lymphoma
    B. Ankylosing spondylitis
    C. Sarcoidosis
    D. Kaposi's sarcoma
    E. Graft versus host reaction

    Answer: D

30. Human immunodeficiency virus can be transmitted from an infected person by all the following routes except:
    A. Heterosexual intercourse
    B. Handshake
    C. Intravenous injection using infected needles
    D. Blood transfusions
    E. Transplacentally from mother to fetus

    Answer: B

31. Amyloid A formed in response to chronic infections is typically deposited in all the following organs except:
    A. Brain
    B. Rectum
    C. Liver
    D. Kidney
    E. Adrenals

    Answer: A

Clinicopathologic Review

Chapter 3—Immunopathology

Symptoms/Findings	Question	Answer
An eye infection was diagnosed in a person who cannot produce tears.	Why are such infections recurrent?	Tears have several functions, such as keeping the cornea and conjunctiva moist. Protective substances, such as lysozyme and IgA, account for the bactericidal action of tears. Without tears, the eyes are prone to recurrent infections.
A child was born without a thymus.	Can this child resist infections?	The thymus is essential for the development of T cells. Children born without a thymus (DiGeorge's syndrome) cannot mount a cell-mediated immune response of the delayed type and cannot efficiently fight infections.
A patient with AIDS had a CD4:CD8 ratio of 0.8.	What is the significance of this finding?	The normal CD4:CD8 ratio, or helper T:suppressor/cytotoxic T cell ratio in peripheral blood is 2.0. Loss of CD4 (helper T) cells is an unfavorable prognostic sign typical of profound immunodeficiency.
IgA was found in a mother's milk.	Is this normal?	Yes. IgA is found in many secretions, including human milk. When ingested, IgA in milk provides immunoprotection to the breastfed baby.
When blood of a potential donor was mixed with the recipient's serum, clumps of RBCs formed at the bottom of the vessel.	Could a blood transfusion be performed safely?	This clumping is called hemagglutination. The recipient's serum contains antibodies to the donor's RBCs. The antibody cross-linked the RBCs and caused them to agglutinate and separate from plasma. Owing to donor-recipient incompatibility, a transfusion should not be performed.

Symptoms/Findings *(con't)*	**Question** *(con't)*	**Answer** *(con't)*
A man experienced attacks of sneezing every spring.	What is the correct diagnosis?	Most likely, these symptoms indicate hay fever. The exact diagnosis can be made by demonstrating hypersensitivity to pollen by skin testing.
Group A blood given to a group B person caused severe hemolysis.	Why did hemolysis occur?	Blood group antigens of the ABO type have corresponding natural antibodies. The RBCs of A blood, when transfused into a B person are hemolyzed by anti-A antibodies. The hemolysis that occurred is typical of a type II hypersensitivity reaction.
Blood and large amounts of protein were found in the urine of a woman with systemic lupus erythematosus (SLE).	What is the explanation for these findings?	SLE is a disease mediated by circulating immune complexes that damage the basement membranes of the glomerulus. The damaged basement membranes are leaky, which accounts for the hematuria and proteinuria (i.e, excretion of RBCs and protein in urine).
When purified protein derivative (PPD) isolated from *Mycobacterium tuberculosis* was injected into the skin of a patient, it induced an area of hardening 1 cm in diameter.	How should this PPD test be interpreted?	PPD, like the bacteria from which it is isolated, can induce granulomas in sensitized persons. A positive test means that the tested person has tuberculosis, or at least was exposed to and infected with *M. tuberculosis*.
A monkey liver was transplanted into a human.	Will the liver survive in the new host?	This is a xenograft, which is transplantation of tissue from one species to another. Xenografts are usually rejected because there are too many antigenic differences between it and the host. Only avascular tissues, such as cornea or cardiac valves, can survive as xenografts.

Copyright © 2000 by W.B. Saunders Company.   All rights reserved.

Symptoms/Findings (con't)	Question (con't)	Answer (con't)
An Rh-positive baby, the second child of an Rh-negative mother, was jaundiced.	Why was the child yellow?	Severe jaundice caused by materno-fetal Rh-incompatibility is typically caused by anti-Rh antibodies produced by an Rh-negative mother previously sensitized to Rh during a prior pregnancy. Sensitization can also occur after abortions or as a result of mismatched blood transfusion with Rh-positive blood.
Proteinuria was detected in a man who had chronic tuberculosis.	What is the explanation for this finding?	The explanation must be sought by kidney biopsy. One possibility is that the kidney is infiltrated with amyloid. Patients with chronic inflammation, such as tuberculosis, may develop systemic amyloidosis (AA type) with symptoms of renal, hepatic, or adrenal dysfunction or insufficiency.

Chapter 4
Neoplasia

Instruction: Match the numbered words or phrases with the most appropriate lettered item. Each lettered item can be used more than once.

- A. Adenoma
- B. Squamous cell carcinoma
- C. Adenocarcinoma
- D. Glioma
- E. Sarcoma

1. Benign tumor of the liver

2. Benign tumor of salivary glands

3. Small polyp of the large intestine

4. Malignant tumor of the sun-exposed skin

5. Malignant tumor of the large intestine composed of neoplastic glands

6. Malignant breast tumor

7. Malignant brain tumor

8. Malignant tumor of fat tissue

9. Malignant tumor originating from striated muscle cells

10. Malignant tumor composed of malignant cartilage cells

    Answers: 1. A, 2. A, 3. A, 4. B, 5. C, 6. C, 7. D, 8. E, 9. E, 10. E

Instruction: Choose the one best answer.

11. A lung tumor that has spread to the brain has metastasized via:
    - A. Lymphatics
    - B. Nerves
    - C. Blood vessels
    - D. Cerebrospinal fluid
    - E. Pleural fluid

    Answer: C

12. Teratomas originate from:
    - A. Germ cells of the ovary
    - B. Brain cells
    - C. Thyroid cells
    - D. Endocrine cells of the pancreas
    - E. Fallopian tubes

    Answer: A

13. Hodgkin's disease is a neoplasm that typically involves the:
    - A. Brain
    - B. Lungs
    - C. Heart
    - D. Liver
    - E. Lymph nodes

    Answer: E

14. Alpha fetoprotein is a tumor marker for malignant tumors originating in the:
    - A. Brain
    - B. Lung
    - C. Liver
    - D. Uterus
    - E. Thyroid

    Answer: C

15. Many tumors secrete their own growth factors. This form of stimulation is called:
    A. Autocrine
    B. Heterocrine
    C. Paracrine
    D. Endocrine
    E. Exocrine

    Answer: A

16. The cancer of chimney sweeps identified in the 18th century in England was related to a component of tar which is chemically classified as:
    A. Polycyclic hydrocarbons
    B. Aflatoxin B1
    C. Azo dyes
    D. Naphthylamine
    E. Arsenic

    Answer: A

17. Workers employed in the chemical industry and exposed to high levels of aniline dyes are at increased risk of developing cancer of the:
    A. Brain
    B. Lung
    C. Stomach
    D. Urinary bladder
    E. Testis

    Answer: D

18. The most important source of chemical carcinogens in the human habitat is:
    A. Cigarette smoke
    B. Asbestos
    C. Air pollution
    D. Food additives
    E. Pesticides in the food

    Answer: A

19. Which of the following physical carcinogens is the cause of most skin cancers in man?
    A. Ultraviolet light
    B. Infra-red light
    C. X-rays
    D. Radon
    E. Gamma rays

    Answer: A

20. Human papillomavirus (HPV) has been implicated in the pathogenesis of carcinoma of the:
    A. Lips
    B. Cervix of the uterus
    C. Liver
    D. Ovaries
    E. Pancreas

    Answer: B

21. Retinoblastoma gene (Rb-1) is classified as a(n):
    A. Oncogene
    B. Tumor suppressor gene
    C. Point mutation
    D. Gene amplification
    E. Viral oncogene inserted into the human genome

    Answer: B

22. Which of the following conditions is characterized by a defect of a DNA repair enzyme?
    A. Neurofibromatosis
    B. Hereditary polyposis coli
    C. Xeroderma pigmentosum
    D. Wilms' tumor
    E. Hodgkin's disease

    Answer: C

23. Carcinoma of the stomach has the highest incidence in:
    A. England
    B. Japan
    C. United States
    D. Israel
    E. France

    Answer: B

24. The incidence of which cancer has been rising in the U.S. during the last 20 years?
    A. Carcinoma of the lung
    B. Carcinoma of the liver
    C. Carcinoma of the stomach
    D. Carcinoma of the thyroid
    E. Malignant brain tumors

    Answer: A

Clinicopathologic Review

Chapter 4—Neoplasia

Symptoms/Findings	Question	Answer
A 60-year-old woman was told by her physician that she has skin cancer.	Will this woman die of skin cancer?	Probably not. Cancer is used to denote all malignant tumors. However, not all malignant tumors are lethal, and many are curable if diagnosed early. Skin cancer is usually diagnosed early and often can be removed in time; thus, most patients can be cured.
A small nodule measuring 2 cm in diameter was removed from the breast of a 25-year-old woman. Even though the nodule appeared encapsulated, it was sent for histologic examination.	Should tumors that, on gross examination, appear benign be examined histologically?	Yes. All tumors should be examined histologically because this is the best way to determine whether a tumor is benign or malignant. A well-circumscribed nodule in the breast of a young woman is most likely a benign fibroadenoma, but one cannot be certain of the diagnosis unless the tumor is examined histologically.
An islet cell tumor measuring 3 cm in diameter was found in the pancreas. There were also metastases in the lymph nodes. On histologic examination, it could not be determined whether the primary tumor was benign or malignant.	Is this tumor benign or malignant?	Malignant. There are numerous features distinguishing benign from malignant tumors. The presence of metastases is the best criterion of malignancy. Even if an islet cell tumor appears to be benign histologically, it should be considered malignant if it has already metastasized.
A 60-year-old woman had basal cell carcinoma of the skin and a meningioma.	Which of these tumors represents the more serious health problem?	Meningioma. Basal cell carcinoma is a skin tumor that has an excellent prognosis and is almost always curable by complete excision. Meningiomas are benign tumors that arise from the meninges enveloping the brain or the spinal cord. These tumors are also curable. However, because of their location, meningiomas may cause serious problems; some of these tumors are located at the base of the brain and may be hard to remove.

Symptoms/Findings (con't)	Question (con't)	Answer (con't)
A 60-year-old man developed lymphoma.	What is the prognosis of this tumor?	Poor. The term *lymphoma* can imply that the tumor is benign, like a fibroma or lipoma. This is not true, however. Lymphoma is actually a colloquial term used for *malignant lymphoma,* a highly malignant tumor. There are no benign lymphomas.
A 14-year-old boy died of osteosarcoma that had metastasized to the lungs.	Where did this tumor most likely arise?	Osteosarcomas, as the name implies, are tumors of bone-forming cells that originate most often in the long bones. Osteosarcomas tend to metastasize by blood (hematogenous metastases), and secondary tumors are usually found in the lungs.
A former shipyard worker who was a smoker developed mesothelioma.	Could this man receive compensation for a workplace-related cancer?	Yes. A considerable number of men working in the shipbuilding industry during World War II were exposed to asbestos and developed lung cancer and mesothelioma. Lung cancer was especially prevalent among those who were also smokers. Lung cancer develops often in smokers who are not exposed to asbestos. However, mesothelioma is almost invariably related to asbestos exposure.
A survivor of the atomic blast in Hiroshima died of leukemia 15 years later.	Could the leukemia have been related to radioactive fallout from the atomic bomb?	Yes. An increased incidence of cancer has been noted among the survivors of the atomic blast in Japan in 1945. Among the tumors that were most commonly related to this event were leukemias, lymphomas, and thyroid tumors. This leukemia was probably caused by irradiation.
The sexual partner of a Japanese man suffering from T-cell leukemia developed the same disease.	Could it be that the leukemia was sexually transmitted?	Yes. Adult T-cell leukemia is caused by the virus HTLV-1. This oncogenic virus is closely related to HIV and can be transmitted from one person to another by blood or body fluids. Sexual transmission has been documented.

Symptoms/Findings *(con't)*	Question *(con't)*	Answer *(con't)*
A woman who was diagnosed as having viral hepatitis B in her youth developed hepatocellular carcinoma at the age of 60 years.	Could the liver tumor be somehow related to the viral hepatitis?	Yes. A high incidence of hepatocellular carcinoma has been noted in parts of the world in which HBV is widespread, and viral hepatitis B is definitely one of the major risk factors for liver cell carcinoma. Many hepatocellular carcinoma cells contain the viral DNA which was integrated into their genome. It is not known why HBV causes liver cancer only in some people. Most persons infected with HBV recover from hepatitis and do not develop cancer.
A 20-year-old man has a father and a brother who have familial polyposis coli and cancer of the large intestine.	Will this man develop colon cancer?	Possibly. Familial polyposis coli (FPC) is inherited as an autosomal dominant trait. Essentially all persons affected by FPC develop invasive cancer. This man has a 50% chance of having inherited the disease. If he has inherited FPC, he will develop cancer.

Chapter 5
Genetic and Developmental Diseases

Instruction: Match the numbered words or phrases with the most appropriate lettered item. Each lettered item can be used more than once.

    A. Autosomal dominant inheritance
    B. Autosomal recessive inheritance
    C. X-linked recessive inheritance
    D. X-linked dominant inheritance
    E. Multifactorial inheritance

1. Anencephaly
2. Meningomyelocele
3. Duchenne's muscular dystrophy
4. Cystic fibrosis
5. Marfan's syndrome
6. Hemophilia A
7. Hemophilia B
8. Fragile X chromosome
9. Diabetes mellitus
10. Familial hypercholesterolemia
11. Tay-Sachs disease
12. Phenylketonuria
13. Lysosomal lipid storage diseases
14. Neurofibromatosis
15. Becker's muscular dystrophy

    Answers: 1. E, 2. E, 3. C, 4. B, 5. A, 6. C, 7. C, 8. C, 9. E, 10. A, 11. B, 12. B, 13. B, 14. A, 15. C

Instruction: Choose the one best answer.

16. Most congenital malformations in humans are:
    A. Of unknown cause
    B. Related to infection during pregnancy
    C. Caused by physical agents
    D. Caused by drugs
    E. Caused by environmental pollution

    Answer: A

17. All the following are considered possible causes of the TORCH syndrome except:
    A. Toxoplasma
    B. Rubella virus
    C. Cytomegalovirus
    D. Herpesvirus
    E. Alcohol

    Answer: E

18. Dilation of lateral ventricles of the brain found in TORCH syndrome is called:
    A. Microphthalmia
    B. Chorioretinitis
    C. Hydrocephalus
    D. Cataract
    E. Vesicles

    Answer: C

19. Trisomy of chromosome 21 is typical of:
    A. Turner's syndrome
    B. Klinefelter's syndrome
    C. Down's syndrome
    D. WAGR (Wilms' tumor, aniridia, genital malformations, mental retardation) syndrome
    E. Congenital retinoblastoma

    Answer: C

20. A male who was tall, slightly effeminate with eunuchoid body proportions and gynecomastia was found to have a 47, XXY karyotype. These findings are typical of:
    A. Turner's syndrome
    B. Klinefelter's syndrome
    C. Fragile X syndrome
    D. Marfan's syndrome
    E. Duchenne's muscular dystrophy

    Answer: B

21. An autosomal dominant trait is characterized by all the following except:
    A. The trait is apparent in heterozygotes
    B. The affected heterozygote has a 50 percent chance of transmitting the gene to each child
    C. The trait is expressed in every generation
    D. The unaffected children of a symptomatic carrier do not transmit the trait
    E. The gene accounting for the trait can be located on any of the 46 chromosomes

    Answer: E

22. Cystic fibrosis may present in newborns with signs of:
    A. Dehydration
    B. Meconium peritonitis
    C. Malabsorption
    D. Diarrhea
    E. Bronchiectasis

    Answer: B

23. The most important complication encountered in persons affected by familial hypercholesterolemia is:
    A. Xanthoma
    B. Atherosclerosis
    C. Fatty liver
    D. Pancreatitis
    E. Subluxation of the lens

    Answer: B

24. The X-linked bleeding disorder caused by a deficiency of factor VIII is called:
    A. Hemophilia A
    B. Hemophilia B
    C. Hemosiderosis
    D. Hemochromatosis
    E. Hemorrhagic fever

    Answer: A

25. Children born with a fragile X chromosome suffer from:
    A. Muscle weakness
    B. Blindness
    C. Spinal cord deformities
    D. Mental retardation
    E. Glucose intolerance

    Answer: D

26. All the following are routinely used in prenatal diagnosis except:
    A. Ultrasound
    B. Chorionic villus biopsy
    C. Fetal skin biopsy
    D. Amniotic fluid analysis
    E. Maternal blood analysis

    Answer: C

27. The most important intracranial complication of the neonatal respiratory syndrome is:
    A. Hydrocephalus
    B. Periventricular hemorrhage possibly expanding into a hematocephalus
    C. Calcification of basal ganglia
    D. Kernicterus
    E. Microcephaly

    Answer: B

28. Sudden infant death syndrome typically occurs:
    A. At the time of birth
    B. During the first few hours after birth
    C. During the first week after birth
    D. During the first month of life
    E. Any time between 2 and 9 months of the first year of life

    Answer: E

Clinicopathologic Review

Chapter 5—Genetic and Developmental Diseases

Symptoms/Findings	Question	Answer
A 22-year-old woman missed her period, but started bleeding 8 weeks after the last menstruation.	What happened?	Most likely, this woman became pregnant and had an early pregnancy that resulted in spontaneous abortion. Most spontaneous abortions occur as a result of congenital abnormalities of the fetus/embryo, and many aborted embryos show chromosomal abnormalities.
A heart murmur was diagnosed in a baby born to a mother who had rubella during the second month of pregnancy.	Is this finding related to the mother's rubella infection?	Most likely. Heart murmurs are common in children, and are not necessarily a sign of congenital heart disease. In view of the maternal rubella infection, however, it would be wise to evaluate this baby's heart further, as rubella embryopathy may cause heart defects.
A child born with ocular defects developed a renal tumor. A chromosomal study revealed chromosomal abnormalities.	What kind of chromosomal changes could one expect?	The congenital syndrome characterized by Wilms' tumor and aniridia is typically associated with the deletion of a segment of chromosome 11. This segment contains the Wilms' tumor suppressor genes and several developmentally important genes, one of which is critical for the development of the iris of the eye.
A mentally retarded child with slanted eyes, epicanthus, and simian crease of the palm was born to a 35-year-old woman.	Could this condition have been diagnosed by prenatal testing?	Yes. This baby most likely has Down's syndrome which can be diagnosed by chromosomal analysis of a specimen obtained by chorionic villus biopsy or amniotic fluid aspiration. Affected children typically have 47 chromosomes, with trisomy of chromosome 21.

Symptoms/Findings *(con't)*	Question *(con't)*	Answer *(con't)*
An infertile 21-year-old woman was found to have a 45,X karyotype.	Since she was postpubertal, did she have male or female secondary sex characteristics?	This woman has Turner's syndrome, which is associated with streak ovaries that do not produce female sex hormones. Therefore, these patients do not develop secondary sex characteristics (breasts, female escutcheon) and do not menstruate.
A man with familial hypercholesterolemia has two sons and two daughters.	How many of his children may also have the disease?	Familial hypercholesterolemia is an autosomal dominant disease. Therefore, every child has a 50% chance to inherit the disease. Theoretically, then, two of the four children could be affected. The risk is equal for both males and females.
A neonate developed meconium ileus shortly after birth.	Do the infant's parents have any signs of this disease?	No. Meconium ileus is a complication of cystic fibrosis. Symptomatic children are homozygous, as symptoms occur only in persons carrying two abnormal alleles. The infant must have inherited one allele from each of his parents who were heterozygous and asymptomatic.
A boy was born to a mother who already had two sons with hemophilia.	Does this boy have hemophilia?	Possibly. Hemophilia is an X-linked recessive disease affecting the sons of asymptomatic carrier females. Each son has a 50% chance of inheriting the disease; thus, this boy could be either affected or not affected.
A woman and a man, both of whom were diabetic, wanted to know whether their unborn child would also be diabetic.	Could this determination be made by prenatal testing?	No. Noninsulin-dependent diabetes is a multifactorial disease that cannot be diagnosed in utero. Approximately 15% of the offspring of diabetic parents develop the disease, but one cannot predict which among these will develop it and which will not.
Parents of an apparently healthy boy who died suddenly during sleep at the age of 4 months were concerned that their second child might die as well.	Is this second child at increased risk for Sudden Infant Death Syndrome (SIDS)?	Yes. Although the cause of SIDS is unknown, the death of one sibling due to SIDS is known to be a definitive risk for subsequent children in that family.

Chapter 6
Fluid and Hemodynamic Disorders

Instruction: Choose the one best answer.

1. All of the following are examples of edema except:
   A. Anasarca
   B. Ascites
   C. Hydrothorax
   D. Hematopericardium
   E. Periorbital swelling

   Answer: D

2. Which of the following is a feature of an exudate but is not typical of a transudate?
   A. Accumulation of fluid in a body cavity
   B. Accumulation of fluid in the alveoli of the lung
   C. Accumulation of fluid in the tissue, with subsequent swelling of the tissue ("tumor")
   D. Accumulation of protein in extracellular spaces
   E. Accumulation of numerous polymorphonuclear leukocytes in extracellular spaces

   Answer: E

3. Oncotic edema caused by reduction of the colloid osmotic pressure of the plasma is a typical feature of chronic failure of the:
   A. Heart
   B. Brain
   C. Lung
   D. Liver
   E. Thyroid

   Answer: D

4. Pulmonary edema is a typical complication of:
   A. Right heart failure
   B. Left heart failure
   C. Pulmonary saddle embolus
   D. Cor pulmonale
   E. Pulmonary fibrosis

   Answer: B

5. Red cheeks in a person who is blushing are an example of:
   A. Hemorrhage
   B. Petechia
   C. Ecchymoses
   D. Active hyperemia
   E. Passive hyperemia

   Answer: D

6. So-called "heart failure cells" found in sputum are caused by:
   A. Right ventricular failure
   B. Left ventricular failure
   C. Cardiac hemorrhage
   D. Aortic hemorrhage
   E. Cyanosis

   Answer: B

7. Arterial hemorrhage can be recognized from venous hemorrhage in that the blood is:
   A. Bright red and flows in a pulsating manner
   B. Dark blue and bluish red and oozing
   C. Greenish and rich in bilirubin
   D. Yellow and rich in bilirubin
   E. Clotting rapidly

   Answer: A

8. Hemoptysis denotes bleeding from the:
   A. Heart
   B. Lungs
   C. Stomach
   D. Large intestine
   E. Kidneys

   Answer: B

9. Melena is a typical complication of:
   A. Rectal ulcer
   B. Gastric ulcer
   C. Skin ulcer
   D. Heart failure
   E. Venous thrombosis

   Answer: B

10. Iron deficiency anemia develops most often due to:
    A. Hematemesis
    B. Hematuria
    C. Metrorrhagia
    D. Hemothorax
    E. Hemopericardium

    Answer: C

11. The proteinaceous meshwork that holds a thrombus together is composed of:
    A. Collagen
    B. Elastic fibers
    C. Fibrin
    D. Fibrinogen
    E. Plasmin

    Answer: C

12. Thrombosis can be initiated by all the following except:
    A. Inflammation
    B. Endothelial cell injury
    C. Stagnation of blood in varicose veins
    D. Hypercoagulability of blood due to shock
    E. Heparin

    Answer: E

13. Marantic nonbacterial or sterile thrombotic endocarditis is characterized by formation of thrombi which are best classified as:
    A. Intramural
    B. Valvular
    C. Arterial
    D. Venous
    E. Capillary

    Answer: B

14. Ingrowth of granulation tissue into a venous thrombus is called:
    A. Conglutination
    B. Sedimentation
    C. Margination
    D. Organization
    E. Infarction

    Answer: D

15. Clinically significant emboli are most often composed of:
    A. Air
    B. Amniotic fluid
    C. Foreign particulate material
    D. Fat
    E. Thrombi

    Answer: E

16. In decompression sickness or caisson disease the emboli are composed of:
    A. Air
    B. Fat
    C. Platelets
    D. Fibrin
    E. Plasminogen

    Answer: A

17. Most venous emboli that are of clinical significance originate in the veins of the:
    A. Lungs
    B. Heart
    C. Kidney
    D. Brain
    E. Lower extremities

    Answer: E

18. Which of the following organs is most affected by venous embolism?
    A. Brain
    B. Heart
    C. Lungs
    D. Liver
    E. Kidneys

    Answer: C

19. Most arterial emboli that cause cerebral infarcts originate from the:
    A. Right ventricle
    B. Left ventricle
    C. Pulmonary artery
    D. Abdominal aorta
    E. Cerebral veins

    Answer: B

20. Red infarcts are typically found in the:
    A. Spleen
    B. Heart
    C. Kidney
    D. Thyroid
    E. Small intestine

    Answer: E

21. Firm fibrous scars are typically found in healed infarcts of all the following organs except the:
    A. Heart
    B. Lung
    C. Spleen
    D. Brain
    E. Kidney

    Answer: D

22. Shock resulting from massive bleeding is best classified as:
    A. Hypotonic
    B. Hypovolemic
    C. Cardiogenic
    D. Neurogenic
    E. Endotoxemic

    Answer: B

23. Waterhouse-Friderichsen syndrome caused by endotoxemic shock is characterized by:
    A. Bleeding into the adrenals and skin
    B. Active hyperemia
    C. Mural thrombi of the left ventricle
    D. Hematoma of the brain
    E. Hypertension

    Answer: A

24. Abscess is a complication of:
    A. Septic embolism
    B. Marantic endocarditis
    C. Air embolism
    D. Fat embolism
    E. Pulmonary saddle embolism

    Answer: A

Clinicopathologic Review

Chapter 6—Fluid and Hemodynamic Disorders

Symptoms/Findings	Question	Answer
A 4-year-old child had a puffy face and brown urine.	What diagnosis do these findings suggest?	This child's abnormal facial edema and brown urine indicate possible kidney disease. Kidney disease leads to loss of protein in the urine, and the consequent hypoproteinemia results in edema.
A 68-year-old man with known heart disease developed pain under the right costal margin.	What is the likely cause of his pain?	Heart failure leads to liver congestion. Expansion of the liver capsule in response to an excess of venous blood stimulates the nerves and is perceived as painful.

Symptoms/Findings *(con't)*	Question *(con't)*	Answer *(con't)*
The sailors who circumnavigated the globe in the 16th century developed bleeding from the gums.	What was the cause of their bleeding?	Bleeding of the gums among ancient mariners during long sea voyages was a consequence of vitamin C deficiency, which caused weakening of the small blood vessels. This is an example of capillary bleeding.
A patient with pulmonary tuberculosis expectorated blood.	What is this called?	Blood in the sputum is called hemoptysis. It is typically caused by rupture of the pulmonary arteries. In tuberculosis, pulmonary blood vessels are typically disrupted by caseous necrosis.
A person with massive traumatic hematoma became jaundiced within 6 days of the injury.	What is the cause of this jaundice?	The blood in hematomas decomposes into bilirubin. Bilirubin from large hematomas may enter the circulation, resulting in jaundice.
A 50-year-old man who presented with sudden chest pain subsequently died.	What findings might the autopsy reveal?	There are many causes of sudden death. In a patient with sudden death and chest pain, one should suspect myocardial infarction. In some of these patients, the autopsy will reveal a fresh thrombus occluding the coronary artery.
A pregnant woman had swollen, painful legs.	What is the cause of swelling?	Many women have circulatory problems during pregnancy that are multifactorial. For example, the enlarged uterus may compress the pelvic veins, causing hydrostatic edema. The blood is also hypercoagulable in pregnancy. Venous stasis and hypercoagulability may cause thrombi of the lower extremities.
A woman with varicose veins developed chest pain and expectorated blood the next day.	What could have caused these symptoms?	Individuals with varicose veins are prone to formation of thrombi which may give rise to emboli. These venous thromboemboli may cause pulmonary infarction. Pain and hemoptysis are symptoms of pulmonary embolism.

Symptoms/Findings *(con't)*	Question *(con't)*	Answer *(con't)*
A 56-year-old man with a prior history of myocardial infarction developed gangrene of the toe.	What is the cause of the gangrene?	In this patient, gangrene is probably attributable to an embolus or thrombus occluding one of the major arteries of the foot. In a patient who has had a previous myocardial infarction, this could also be related to an embolus originating from the mural endocardium overlying the infarcted left ventricle.
A person with burn injuries became short of breath. Auscultation revealed pulmonary rales.	What is the likely diagnosis?	This person most likely has pulmonary edema, which is the first sign of ARDS. Burns lead to fluid loss and cause hypovolemic shock. In this patient, pulmonary edema could also be caused by thermal injury of the pulmonary respiratory epithelium.

Chapter 7
The Cardiovascular System

Instruction: Match the numbered words or phrases with the most appropriate lettered item. Each lettered item can be used more than once.

- A. Congenital heart disease
- B. Ischemic vascular disease
- C. Hypertension-related disease
- D. Inflammatory disease
- E. Metabolic disease

1. Tetralogy of Fallot

2. Maternal rubella infection during pregnancy

3. Myocardial infarct

4. Rheumatic fever

5. Interventricular septal defect

6. Thrombotic cerebrovascular accident complicating atherosclerosis

7. Stroke in a person with chronic renal disease

8. Hyperlipidemia

9. Angina pectoris

10. Bacterial endocarditis

Answers: 1. A, 2. A, 3. B, 4. D, 5. A, 6. B, 7. C, 8. E, 9. B, 10. D

Instruction: Choose the one best answer.

11. Which is the most common congenital heart defect recognized in clinical practice?
    - A. Interatrial septal defect
    - B. Interventricular septal defect
    - C. Tetralogy of Fallot
    - D. Transposition of great vessels
    - E. Coarctation of the aorta

    Answer: B

12. All the following are risk factors of atherosclerosis except:
    - A Advanced age
    - B. Heredity
    - C. Diabetes
    - D. Hypertension
    - E. Estrogens

    Answer: E

13. Which of the following has been implicated in pathogenesis of atherosclerosis?
    - A. Regular exercise
    - B. Alcohol
    - C. Cigarette smoking
    - D. Aspirin
    - E. Antihypertensive drugs

    Answer: C

14. Atherosclerotic aneurysms are most often located in:
    - A. Coronary arteries
    - B. Ascending aorta
    - C. Thoracic aorta
    - D. Abdominal aorta
    - E. Iliac arteries

    Answer: D

15. Atherosclerotic narrowing of which artery causes hypertension?
    A. Middle cerebral artery
    B. Anterior descending branch of the left coronary artery
    C. Right coronary artery
    D. Renal artery
    E. Femoral artery

    Answer: D

16. Intermittent claudication is caused by atherosclerosis of:
    A. Carotid artery
    B. Subclavian artery
    C. Splenic artery
    D. Renal artery
    E. Popliteal artery

    Answer: E

17. Infarction of the posterior half of the interventricular septum is caused by an occlusion of the:
    A. Main trunk of the left coronary artery
    B. Anterior descending branch of the left coronary artery
    C. Circumflex branch of the left coronary artery
    D. Right coronary artery
    E. Coronary sinus

    Answer: D

18. Acute cardiac tamponade is typically a complication of:
    A. Rupture of the left ventricle due to myocardial infarction
    B. Mural thrombosis
    C. Ventricular aneurysm
    D. Subendocardial circumferential myocardial infarction
    E. Rupture of the papillary muscle

    Answer: A

19. Myocardial infarction is accompanied by typical biochemical changes. Elevation of which enzyme in the blood occurs first following the occlusion of a coronary artery?
    A. Alanine aminotransferase
    B. Aspartate aminotransferase
    C. Creatine kinase
    D. Lactate dehydrogenase
    E. Acid phosphatase

    Answer: C

20. The most common form of arterial hypertension is considered to be:
    A. Essential or idiopathic
    B. Caused by kidney disease
    C. Caused by adrenal cortical hyperactivity
    D. Secondary to adrenal medullar tumors
    E. Secondary to the narrowing of the aorta

    Answer: A

21. Rheumatic carditis is typically preceded by:
    A. Streptococcal throat infection
    B. Staphylococcal skin infection
    C. Gonococcal arthritis
    D. Coxsackie B virus myositis
    E. Influenza

    Answer: A

22. The most common complication of rheumatic endocarditis is:
    A. Bacterial endocarditis
    B. Viral endocarditis
    C. Fungal myocarditis
    D. Parasitic endocarditis
    E. Pulmonary embolism

    Answer: A

23. The most common cause of infectious myocarditis in the U.S. is:
    A. Toxoplasma gondii
    B. Trypanosoma cruzi
    C. Coxsackie B virus
    D. Treponema pallidum
    E. Streptococcus pneumoniae

    Answer: C

24. All the following represent iatrogenic heart lesions except:
    A. Alcoholic cardiomyopathy
    B. Radiation-induced heart disease
    C. Doxorubicin-induced heart disease
    D. Digitalis toxicity
    E. Postcardiotomy pericarditis

    Answer: A

Clinicopathologic Review

Chapter 7—The Cardiovascular System

Symptoms/Findings	Question	Answer
A 2-year-old child had bluish lips and fingers and appeared short of breath. Congenital heart failure was diagnosed.	Why do children with congestive heart failure develop cyanosis?	Cyanosis is bluish discoloration of the skin that develops because the blood contains more than 5 g/mL of unsaturated hemoglobin. In congenital heart failure, cyanosis develops owing to the mixing of unoxygenated venous blood with the arterial blood in the left ventricle secondary to right-to-left shunt.
A 30-year-old man was told that he had a heart murmur.	What produces heart murmurs?	Heart murmurs are caused by blood passing through pathologically altered orifices between the atria and ventricles or between the ventricles and the pulmonary artery and the aorta. The type of heart murmur depends on the underlying pathologic process which may result in valvular stenosis or incompetence.
"Heart block" was diagnosed by EKG in a 70-year-old man.	What causes heart block?	The regular action of the heart depends on the normal conductance of electric stimuli from the sinoatrial node to the atrioventricular node and then through the conduction system into the ventricle. The interruption of this normal sequence is most often caused by ischemia. Heart block is a feature of coronary heart disease.
A 50-year-old man complained of chest pain.	What is the significance of precordial pain?	Chest pain that is anterior to the heart (precordial pain) is caused by myocardial ischemia, which is typical of coronary heart disease. The chest pain is an early sign of impending infarct, but not all chest pains are caused by heart disease.

Copyright © 2000 by W.B. Saunders Company. All rights reserved.

Symptoms/Findings *(con't)*	Question *(con't)*	Answer *(con't)*
A 55-year-old woman was diagnosed as having angina pectoris.	What is angina pectoris?	In Latin, this term means chest pain. In clinical medicine, the term refers to precordial pain that typically occurs during exercise or strain. It is caused by insufficient blood supply to the heart secondary to narrowing of the coronary artery. Anginal pain responds well to vasodilators, such as nitroglycerin.
A 50-year-old man complained of shortness of breath.	Why do patients with cardiac disease often have shortness of breath?	Congestive heart failure results in inadequate perfusion of the lungs or pulmonary congestion and edema. Because the blood is not adequately oxygenated in the lungs, these patients have a "craving for oxygen" and often become short of breath.
A 60-year-old man complained of leg cramps which were so severe that he had to stop walking.	What causes intermittent claudication?	Narrowing of the arteries of the legs secondary to atherosclerosis causes ischemia of the muscles. When a person walks, the ischemia worsens because active muscles need increased amounts of oxygen. Cramping results, which may be so severe that the patient must discontinue walk.

Chapter 8
The Respiratory System

Instruction: Match the numbered words or phrases with the most appropriate lettered item. Each lettered item can be used more than once.

    A. Infectious disease
    B. Immune disease
    C. Mineral dust-induced disease
    D. Circulatory disease
    E. Tumor

1. Carcinoid
2. Mesothelioma
3. Asthma
4. Croup
5. Lobar pneumonia
6. Bronchiectasis
7. Legionnaire's disease
8. Ghon complex
9. Sarcoidosis
10. Pneumoconiosis
11. Silicosis
12. Asbestosis

Answers: 1. E, 2. E, 3. B, 4. A, 5. A, 6. A, 7. A, 8. A, 9. B, 10. C, 11. C, 12. C

Instruction: Choose the one best answer.

13. The most common of all the infections of the respiratory tract is:
    A. Upper respiratory infection
    B. Laryngitis
    C. Tracheitis
    D. Pneumonia
    E. Pleuritis

    Answer: A

14. Bronchiolitis of children is in most instances caused by:
    A. Bacteria
    B. Viruses
    C. Fungi
    D. Parasites
    E. *Pneumocystis carinii*

    Answer: B

15. Lung infection that develops in patients who have heart failure and pulmonary edema is called:
    A. Interstitial pneumonia
    B. Hypostatic pneumonia
    C. Bronchiectasis
    D. Chronic obstructive pulmonary disease
    E. Lobar pneumonia

    Answer: B

16. Mycoplasma pneumoniae infection usually causes:
    A. Lobar pneumonia
    B. Lobular pneumonia
    C. Aspiration pneumonia
    D. Interstitial pneumonia
    E. Abscesses

    Answer: D

17. Miliary tuberculosis is characterized by:
    A. Granuloma formation
    B. Abscess formation
    C. Lobar pneumonia
    D. Acute bronchitis
    E. Acute bronchiolitis

    Answer: A

18. The major pulmonary complication of congenital alpha-1-antitrypsin deficiency is:
    A. Chronic bronchitis
    B. Bronchiectasis
    C. Atelectasis
    D. Emphysema
    E. Mesothelioma

    Answer: D

19. The most important cause of emphysema is:
    A. Cigarette smoking
    B. Air pollution in the cities
    C. Tuberculosis
    D. AIDS
    E. Asthma

    Answer: A

20. Attacks of intrinsic asthma may be precipitated by all the following except:
    A. Exercise
    B. Bronchial infection
    C. Aspirin
    D. Corticosteroids
    E. Psychological stress

    Answer: D

21. In lungs affected by sarcoidosis there are numerous granulomas and infiltrates of:
    A. T-suppressor lymphocytes
    B. T-helper lymphocytes
    C. B lymphocytes
    D. Eosinophils
    E. Plasma cells

    Answer: B

22. Coal-worker's lung disease is best classified as:
    A. Asbestosis
    B. Pneumoconiosis
    C. Acute hypersensitivity reaction
    D. Chronic hypersensitivity reaction
    E. Chronic bacterial pneumonitis

    Answer: B

23. All the following lung lesions have been linked to asbestos exposure except:
    A. Bronchial asthma
    B. Pulmonary fibrosis
    C. Pleural fibrosis and plaques
    D. Lung cancer
    E. Mesothelioma

    Answer: A

24. Fibrin-rich hyaline membranes and protein-rich intra-alveolar edema are features of:
    A. Atelectasis
    B. Diffuse alveolar damage (DAD) in adult respiratory distress syndrome (ARDS)
    C. Emphysema
    D. Bronchiectasis
    E. Aspiration pneumonia

    Answer: B

25. Approximately 90% of all patients with lung cancer present with a history of:
    A. Alcoholism
    B. Hereditary cancer syndromes
    C. Cigarette smoking
    D. Exposure to chemical carcinogens in food and water
    E. Obesity

    Answer: C

26. The most common presenting symptom of lung cancer is:
    A. Prolonged coughing and expectoration
    B. Bleeding
    C. Chest pain
    D. Pleural effusion
    E. Hoarseness due to nerve paralysis

    Answer: A

27. Pleural tumors are usually associated with:
    A. Pneumothorax
    B. Hemothorax
    C. Pyothorax
    D. Pleural effusion
    E. Empyema

    Answer: D

Clinicopathologic Review

Chapter 8—The Respiratory System

Symptoms/Findings	Question	Answer
A young man sneezed each time he was close to cats.	What is the cause of his sneezing?	This man is probably allergic to cats and has developed an allergic rhinitis. Although popularly called hay fever, it may be caused by many other allergens besides hay and grass pollen.
A 3-year-old with hay fever and barking cough was brought to the hospital in respiratory distress.	What is this child's diagnosis?	This child has "croup," or acute laryngitis. The narrowing of the airway tube is caused by an acute infection, which is usually viral.
A 50-year-old chronic alcoholic was brought to the hospital with fever and shortness of breath. He was coughing and expectorating yellow sputum.	What is the most likely cause of his distress?	Alcoholics and other people whose natural resistance is reduced are prone to pneumonia. Fever, shortness of breath, and purulent sputum are highly suggestive of pneumonia. The diagnosis should be confirmed by chest x-ray examination.
A medical student who felt ill developed a low-grade fever. She was found to have a pleural effusion.	What is the explanation for these findings?	Pleural effusion that is associated with mild, nonspecific symptoms is not diagnostic of any specific disease. Hydrothorax in young people is usually secondary to inflammation. Viral and mycoplasmal infection and tuberculosis should be high on the list of possible causes. Transudate secondary to heart failure and carcinomatous effusions are less likely. A sample of the pleural fluid should be obtained and analyzed to determine the final diagnosis.

Symptoms/Findings *(con't)*	Question *(con't)*	Answer *(con't)*
A chronic smoker who was admitted to the hospital had shortness of breath and expectorating large amounts of yellowish sputum. There was no fever or leg edema.	What is the diagnosis?	Shortness of breath may be caused by pulmonary or cardiac problems. In a chronic smoker with a productive, mucopurulent cough, the most likely diagnosis is chronic bronchitis and emphysema, which produce symptoms of chronic lung disease.
A 5-year-old child has an attack of suffocating cough accompanied by wheezing respiration. There was no fever, but the child appeared anxious and in distress.	What is the diagnosis?	Sudden onset of cough with wheezing indicates bronchospasm. Most likely, this is an attack of asthma, which can be effectively treated with appropriate medication.
In an asthmatic child, clinical tests showed a sensitivity to cat dandruff. Blood studies were also performed.	Which finding would support the diagnosis of asthma?	Asthmatic children often show an increased number of eosinophils in the differential white blood count of peripheral blood. One might detect an elevated plasma IgE level. However, the diagnosis of asthma is made primarily on the basis of clinical finding.
A 60-year-old coal miner developed progressive shortness of breath, and the x-ray studies showed numerous nodular masses in both lungs.	What diagnoses should be considered?	This patient could have one of several pathologic processes that affect coal workers. The most likely is anthracosilicosis, which typically produces nodular masses that are visible on radiography. These workers are also prone to tuberculosis.
A 35-year-old man was salvaged from a burning house. Because of marked shortness of breath, he was placed on a ventilator.	What is the cause of the shortness of breath?	The patient is either in hypovolemic shock because he has lost fluid through the skin burns, or he has suffered lung damage from inhalation of hot air and toxic fumes. All of these conditions can cause ARDS. Respiratory distress is secondary to pulmonary intra-alveolar edema or a loss of normal alveolar respiratory surfaces, or both.

Symptoms/Findings *(con't)*	Question *(con't)*	Answer *(con't)*
A chronic smoker became hoarse and, after a few days, could not speak at all.	What is the appropriate course of action for this patient?	Chronic smokers are at risk of developing cancer of the larynx. Tumors of the vocal cords typically present with hoarseness or loss of voice (aphonia). These patients should be referred to an otorhinolaryngologist for laryngoscopic examination. If carcinoma is diagnosed, it should be resected surgically.
A chronic smoker with a long-standing chronic bronchitis expectorated blood during a paroxysm of coughing.	What is the cause of the hemoptysis?	Hemoptysis, or blood in the sputum, can have many causes. The straining with coughing that accompanies chronic bronchitis may lead to rupture of bronchial vessels and bleeding. However, the physician should also consider the possibility that this man has developed cancer. Cancer is a well-known cause of hemoptysis.
During a routine chest x-ray examination in a 60-year-old woman, three round nodules were found in the left lung and two in the right lung.	What is the most likely diagnosis?	Round "cannonball" lesions seen on x-ray studies are most likely metastatic tumors. A biopsy must be performed to confirm the diagnosis, and a clinical examination should be performed to determine the site of the primary tumor.

Chapter 9
The Hematopoietic and Lymphoid System

Instruction: Match the numbered words or phrases with the most appropriate lettered item. Each lettered item can be used more than once.

    A.   Disease of red blood cells and their precursors
    B.   Disease of segmented leukocytes and their precursors
    C.   Disease of lymphocytes and their precursors and descendants
    D.   Disease of platelets and megakaryocytes
    E.   Disease of soluble clotting factors

1. Hemophilia A
2. Thrombocytopenia
3. Iron deficiency anemia
4. Acute myelogenous leukemia
5. Acute lymphoblastic leukemia
6. Hodgkin's disease
7. Multiple myeloma
8. Idiopathic thrombocytopenic purpura
9. Bleeding tendency due to vitamin K deficiency
10. Neutropenia (agranulocytosis)
11. Megaloblastic anemia
12. Sickle cell anemia
13. Thalassemia minor
14. Hereditary spherocytosis
15. Polycythemia
16. Burkitt's lymphoma

Answers: 1. E, 2. D, 3. A, 4. B, 5. C, 6. C, 7. C, 8. D, 9. E, 10. B, 11. A, 12. A, 13. A, 14. A, 15. A, 16. C

Instruction: Choose the one best answer.

17. Microcytic hypochromic anemia with low hemosiderin stores in the bone marrow will respond favorably to treatment with:
    A.   Vitamin C
    B.   Vitamin B_{12}
    C.   Folic acid
    D.   Iron
    E.   Selenium
Answer: D

18. Macrocytic, megaloblastic anemia occurs typically in association with:
    A.   Chronic dermatitis
    B.   Atrophic gastritis
    C.   Hypothyroidism
    D.   Old age
    E.   Chronic osteoarthritis
Answer: B

19. Aplastic anemia is most often:
    A.   Idiopathic
    B.   Secondary to viral infection
    C.   Radiation induced
    D.   Drug induced
    E.   Immune mediated
Answer: A

20. All of the following are hemolytic anemias caused by red blood cell abnormalities (intracorpuscular defects) except:
    A. Sickle cell anemia
    B. Hereditary spherocytosis
    C. Thalassemia major
    D. Thalassemia minor
    E. Autoimmune hemolytic anemia

    Answer: E

21. The sickling of red blood cells of patients with sickle cell anemia can be induced in vitro by adding:
    A. Normal blood
    B. Normal serum
    C. Oxygen
    D. Oxygen-binding chemical such as metabisulfite
    E. Alkali

    Answer: D

22. Sickle cell hemoglobin is routinely identified in the laboratory by:
    A. Polarized light microscopy
    B. Electron microscopy
    C. Electrophoresis
    D. Immunochemistry
    E. Electron spin microscopy

    Answer: C

23. Thalassemia minor is a disease involving the gene that encodes:
    A. Globin chains of hemoglobin
    B. The heme portion of hemoglobin
    C. The iron-binding portion of hemoglobin
    D. The porphyrin ring of hemoglobin
    E. Bilirubin synthetase

    Answer: A

24. All the following findings are typical of secondary polycythemia except:
    A. Increased number of red blood cells in circulation
    B. Hyperviscosity of the blood
    C. Increased number of erythroid precursors in the bone marrow
    D. Increased incidence of thrombi
    E. Association with myelodysplastic syndromes

    Answer: E

25. Epstein-Barr virus, a possible cause of Burkitt's lymphoma, has a predilection for infecting:
    A. T-suppressor/cytotoxic lymphocytes
    B. T-helper lymphocytes
    C. Plasma cells
    D. B lymphocytes
    E. Eosinophils

    Answer: D

26. Which virus is a proven cause of leukemia/lymphoma in humans?
    A. E-B virus
    B. HIV
    C. HTLV-1
    D. HPV
    E. CMV

    Answer: C

27. Overall the most common form of leukemia is:
    A. Acute lymphoblastic leukemia
    B. Acute myelogenous leukemia
    C. Chronic lymphocytic leukemia
    D. Chronic myelogenous leukemia
    E. Plasma cell leukemia

    Answer: B

28. The most common form of leukemia in children under the age of 5 years is:
    A. Acute lymphoblastic leukemia
    B. Acute myelogenous leukemia
    C. Chronic lymphocytic leukemia
    D. Chronic myelogenous leukemia
    E. Plasma cell leukemia

    Answer: A

29. Which of the following leukemias has the best prognosis without chemotherapy?
    A. Acute lymphoblastic leukemia
    B. Acute myelogenous leukemia
    C. Chronic lymphocytic leukemia
    D. Chronic myelogenous leukemia
    E. Plasma cell leukemia

    Answer: C

30. The most common symptom of lymphomas is:
    A. Lymph node enlargement
    B. Infection
    C. Fever
    D. Pruritus
    E. Sweating

    Answer: A

31. Which of the following lymphomas is classified as a low-grade lymphoma?
    A. Follicular lymphoma
    B. Diffuse large cell lymphoma
    C. Burkitt's lymphoma
    D. Immunoblastic lymphoma
    E. Lymphoblastic lymphoma

    Answer: A

32. The diagnostic feature of multiple myeloma is best documented by:
    A. Peripheral blood smear analysis
    B. Serum electrophoresis
    C. Measurement of serum osmolarity
    D. Measurement of serum calcium
    E. Molecular biology

    Answer: B

33. Punched-out bone lesions of the calvaria seen by x-ray examination are typical of:
    A. Hodgkin's disease
    B. Thrombotic thrombocytopenic purpura
    C. Multiple myeloma
    D. Aplastic anemia
    E. Lymphocytic lymphoma

    Answer: C

34. Consumption of platelets associated with widespread hemorrhages is a feature of:
    A. Hemophilia A
    B. Hemophilia B
    C. Aplastic anemia
    D. Leukemia
    E. Disseminated intravascular coagulopathy (DIC)

    Answer: E

35. Fibrin-split-products are typically found in the urine of patients who have:
    A. Hemophilia A
    B. Hemophilia B
    C. Disseminated intravascular coagulation (DIC)
    D. Aplastic anemia
    E. Thrombocytopenia

    Answer: C

Clinicopathologic Review

Chapter 9—The Hematopoietic and Lymphoid Systems

Symptoms/Findings	Question	Answers
A 20-year-old woman with pale skin and conjunctiva reported chronic fatigue. Her hematocrit level was 35.	What is the cause of her symptoms?	Anemia causes fatigue, and the skin and mucosa of affected persons will appear pale. In a young menstruating woman, the most common cause of these findings is iron deficiency anemia.
A 40-year-old man was found to have a low red blood cell count, low mean corpuscular volume (MCV), and low mean corpuscular hemoglobin concentration (MCHC).	What is the diagnosis?	Anemia that is associated with low MCV and MCHC is considered to be microcytic hypochromic anemia, and is typically caused by iron deficiency. In males, it is often a sign of chronic blood loss (e.g., from a peptic ulcer).

Symptoms/Findings *(con't)*	Question *(con't)*	Answer *(con't)*
A pregnant woman presented with a low red blood cell count and a high MCV.	What is the diagnosis and most likely cause of this condition?	This pregnant woman has macrocytic anemia. Most likely, it is attributable to a relative folic acid deficiency caused by the increased demand for this vitamin in pregnancy.
A 12-year-old boy with sickle cell anemia developed pain in the hip.	What is the cause of this symptom?	This patient most likely developed a sickling crisis, which led to an occlusion of blood vessels and ischemic necrosis of the bone.
A 3-year-old child was found to have numerous bleeding sites.	What is the likely cause of this bleeding?	There are numerous causes of bleeding. Nevertheless, if the bleeding is extensive one should exclude leukemia. Leukemic cells infiltrate the bone marrow and destroy the megakaryocytes, which leads to thrombocytopenia and uncontrollable bleeding.
Recurrent pneumonia was reported in a 50-year-old man who also had profuse bleeding of the gums.	What could be the cause of these findings?	Recurrent infections indicate reduced resistance to disease, the possible causes of which are numerous. Peripheral blood examination may yield some clues. Most notably, it is important to exclude AIDS, aplastic anemia, and leukemia, which could cause bone marrow failure and these symptoms.
Enlarged lymph nodes were noted in the groin axilla of a 55-year-old woman.	What is the most likely diagnosis?	Lymph node enlargement can accompany infection. Widespread lymphadenopathy that does not subside should be examined further and the diagnosis of lymphoma should be excluded by lymph node biopsy.

Symptoms/Findings (con't)	Question (con't)	Answer (con't)
A 50-year-old man who reported pain under the left costal margin was found to have an enlarged spleen on palpation.	What is the cause of his splenic enlargement?	There are many causes of splenomegaly, including circulatory congestive splenomegaly associated with liver cirrhosis and infectious splenomegaly associated with congenital errors of metabolism (e.g., in Gaucher's disease). It is important to remember that leukemia and lymphoma also cause splenomegaly. These diseases should, therefore, be excluded in this patient.
Knee stiffening and immobility developed in 30-year-old hemophiliac.	What is the cause of this symptom?	Hemophiliacs are prone to bleeding into the joints. Hemarthrosis is a common symptom, and if it recurs many times, it may cause structural disturbances in the joint, including joint stiffness and an inability to walk.

Chapter 10
The Gastrointestinal System

Instruction: Match the numbered words or phrases with the most appropriate lettered item. Each lettered item can be used more than once.

    A. Infectious disease
    B. Multifactorial disease or disease of unknown etiology
    C. Acquired obstructive disorder affecting the passage of food
    D. Developmental or genetic disorder
    E. Neoplasm

1. Hirschsprung's disease
2. Pseudomembranous colitis
3. Celiac sprue
4. Crohn's disease
5. Ulcerative colitis
6. Diverticulosis of the colon
7. Atrophic gastritis
8. Peptic ulcer
9. Periodontal disease
10. Achalasia
11. Linitis plastica
12. Acute appendicitis
13. Ileus
14. Peritonitis
15. Inguinal hernia
16. Intussusception
17. Volvulus
18. Whipple's disease
19. Adenomatous polyp of the colon (tubular adenoma)
20. Peutz-Jeghers polyps

Answers: 1. D, 2. A, 3. B, 4. B, 5. B, 6. C, 7. B, 8. B, 9. A, 10. C, 11. E, 12. A, 13. C, 14. A, 15. C, 16. C, 17. C, 18. A, 19. E, 20. D

Instruction: Choose the one best answer.

21. Dental caries begins by the formation of:
    A. Pockets of periodontal inflammation
    B. Bacterial plaques on the surface of the tooth
    C. Periapical granuloma
    D. Periapical abscess
    E. Radicular cyst

Answer: B

22. Atrophic gastritis is characterized by:
    A. Xerostomia
    B. Achlorhydria
    C. Gastric hyperacidity
    D. Achalasia
    E. Reflux esophagitis

Answer: B

23. Carcinoma of the oral cavity presenting as a white, slightly elevated plaque is clinically described as:
    A. Leukoplakia
    B. Erythroplakia
    C. Ulcer
    D. Crater
    E. Nodule

    Answer: A

24. The most common viral cause of sialadenitis is:
    A. Herpesvirus
    B. Measles virus
    C. Mumps virus
    D. Cytomegalovirus
    E. Epstein-Barr virus

    Answer: C

25. The most common tumor of the salivary glands is:
    A. Pleomorphic adenoma
    B. Adenoid cystic carcinoma
    C. Mucoepidermoid carcinoma
    D. Adenocarcinoma of major ducts
    E. Squamous cell carcinoma

    Answer: A

26. Peptic esophagitis is caused by:
    A. Exogenous acids in food
    B. Spices
    C. Viruses
    D. Fungi
    E. Reflux of gastric juice

    Answer: E

27. Most malignant tumors of the esophagus are histologically classified as:
    A. Adenocarcinoma
    B. Transitional cell carcinoma
    C. Small-cell carcinoma
    D. Squamous cell carcinoma
    E. Sarcomas

    Answer: D

28. All the following are common symptoms and/or complications of duodenal ulcer except:
    A. Hematemesis
    B. Melena
    C. Vomiting
    D. Epigastric pain
    E. Carcinoma

    Answer: E

29. Diverticula of the intestine are most often located in the:
    A. Jejunum
    B. Ileum
    C. Cecum
    D. Transverse colon
    E. Sigmoid colon

    Answer: E

30. The changes typical of Crohn's disease are found most often in the:
    A. Anus
    B. Rectum
    C. Sigmoid colon
    D. Transverse colon
    E. Terminal ileum

    Answer: E

31. Crypt abscesses, serpiginous ulcerations, inflammatory polyps of the large intestine are typical features of:
    A. Diverticulosis coli
    B. Crohn's disease
    C. Ulcerative colitis
    D. Pseudomembranous colitis
    E. Cholera

    Answer: C

32. Bacteriologically sterile peritonitis is a complication of:
    A. Ruptured gastric ulcer
    B. Gangrene of the large intestine
    C. Gonococcal salpingitis
    D. Acute pancreatitis
    E. Acute appendicitis

    Answer: D

33. Obstructive ileus may be caused by all the following except:
    A. Gallstones
    B. Fecaliths
    C. Volvulus
    D. Incarceration of intestinal loops in a hernia sac
    E. Spinal cord injury

    Answer: E

34. Which of the following diseases causing malabsorption is associated with diagnostic pathologic changes in the intestine?
    A. Diabetes
    B. Radiation enteritis
    C. Pancreatic insufficiency
    D. Celiac sprue
    E. Intestinal bacterial overgrowth

    Answer: D

35. Genetic predisposition to colonic cancer is inherited as an autosomal dominant trait in:
    A. Hirschsprung's disease
    B. Familial adenomatous polyposis syndrome
    C. Peutz-Jeghers syndrome
    D. Colonic diverticulosis
    E. Ulcerative colitis

    Answer: B

36. Most pedunculated colonic neoplastic polyps are classified as:
    A. Hyperplastic polyp
    B. Juvenile polyp
    C. Inflammatory polyp
    D. Tubular adenoma
    E. Villous adenoma

    Answer: D

37. Approximately 50 percent of all carcinomas of the intestine develop in the:
    A. Rectosigmoid area
    B. Descending colon
    C. Transverse colon
    D. Ascending colon
    E. Small intestine

    Answer: A

38. The best serologic marker of colonic carcinoma is:
    A. Alpha fetoprotein
    B. Carcinoembryonic antigen
    C. Chorionic gonadotropin
    D. Alkaline phosphatase
    E. Acid phosphatase

    Answer: B

Clinicopathologic Review

Chapter 10—The Gastrointestinal System

Symptoms/Findings	Question	Answer
A 20-year-old man visited the dentist because of throbbing pain in the lower jaw.	Is this typical of caries?	Caries (literally meaning rotting of teeth) can present with pain. However, throbbing pain usually reflects an accumulation of pus within the dental pulp (purulent pulpitis) or extension of inflammation in the periodontal tissue, where it may form a periodontal abscess.

Symptoms/Findings *(con't)*	Question *(con't)*	Answer *(con't)*
Painful superficial ulcers developed in the mouth of a 14-year-old girl.	What is the diagnosis?	Most likely, these lesions are canker sores. The causes of aphthous stomatitis, as these sores are known, remain obscure, but usually, the mucosal defects heal on their own, without residual consequences.
A 30-year-old woman had enlarged parotid glands and dry mouth and eyes.	What is the most likely diagnosis?	Xerostomia (dry mouth) and xerophthalmia (dry eyes) with enlargement of salivary glands is typical of Sjögren's syndrome. This autoimmune disease is associated with lymphocytic infiltrates of salivary and lacrimal glands which cause their enlargement. Destruction of the parenchymal cells affects their function and results in decreased production of saliva and tears.
A 40-year-old man had retrosternal pain that was most pronounced when lying down after meals. This was associated with regurgitation of gastric acid into his mouth.	What is the cause of his pain?	Retrosternal (midline chest) pain may be caused by many diseases. However, if associated with regurgitation of gastric contents, it is most likely caused by reflux esophagitis. This could be a consequence of lower esophageal sphincter insufficiency or hiatal hernia, or some esophageal motility problem.
A 60-year-old man with a history of heavy smoking and alcohol consumption could not swallow meat.	What should be done?	First one must determine the cause of dysphagia. This can be done by endoscopy or by x-ray examination following barium swallow. Dysphagia can be caused by functional disturbances of esophageal motility, but it may also be a symptom of esophageal cancer.
A 40-year-old man complained of epigastric pain 3 to 4 hours after meals. He could pinpoint the most painful site on the anterior abdominal wall.	What is the diagnosis?	Most likely, this man has a duodenal peptic ulcer. The diagnosis can be confirmed by endoscopy or x-ray examination with barium swallow. Peptic ulcers usually respond favorably to drug treatment.

Symptoms/Findings *(con't)*	Question *(con't)*	Answer *(con't)*
A 60-year-old man complained of weight loss, weakness, vomiting, and nausea and then noted enlarged nodes on the left side of his neck.	What should be done?	A biopsy sample of the neck node should be obtained especially in a patient with symptoms that could be related to cancer. If the lymph node biopsy shows adenocarcinoma, there is a high probability that the patient has gastric cancer. Supraclavicular lymph nodes are a common extra-abdominal site of metastasis of gastric cancer.
A 20-year-old woman complained of frequent bowel movements and bloody stools.	What is the diagnosis?	As bloody diarrhea is a symptom of many diseases, the diagnosis cannot be made on the basis of history alone. Additional tests should, therefore, be performed. These include endoscopy to determine which part of the intestine is involved, and culture of the stool sample for bacteria, amoebas, or other pathogens. If the symptoms persist and no cause is established, one must consider the possibility of Crohn's disease or ulcerative colitis, and a biopsy of the affected intestine should be performed.
A 60-year-old man reported having pencil-like stools that were tinged with blood.	What should be done?	These findings are highly suggestive of cancer of the left side of the colon. Rectal examination can detect at least one third of all tumors. If the tumor is not palpated, a rectoscopic or (even deeper) colonoscopic examination should be performed to determine the site of obstruction.

Chapter 11
The Liver and Biliary Tract

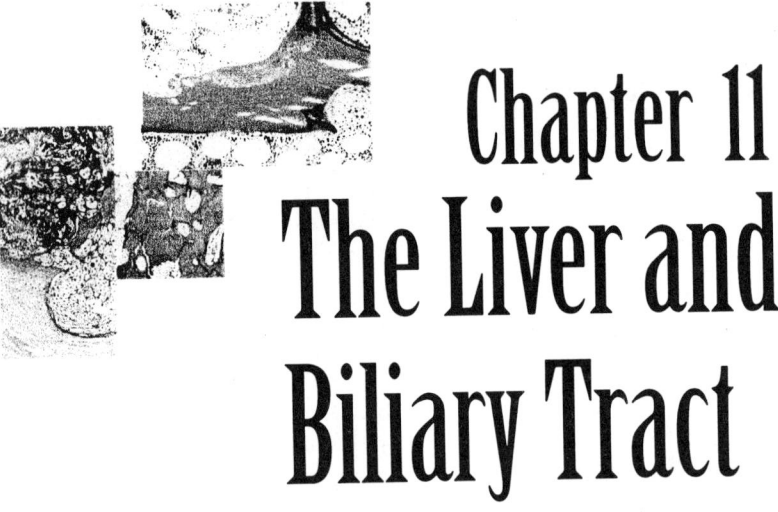

Instruction: Choose the one best answer.

1. All the following are major functions of the liver except:
   A. Excretory
   B. Metabolic
   C. Storage
   D. Neuroendocrine
   E. Synthetic

   Answer: D

2. The nutrients reach the liver from the intestine through the:
   A. Splenic vein
   B. Vena cava inferior
   C. Vena cava superior
   D. Portal vein
   E. Hepatic vein

   Answer: D

3. The lack of bile adversely affects the absorption of all the following vitamins except:
   A. Vitamin A
   B. Vitamin B_{12}
   C. Vitamin K
   D. Vitamin D
   E. Vitamin B

   Answer: B

4. Which of the following serum enzymes is the most reliable marker of extrahepatic biliary obstruction?
   A. Alanine aminotransferase
   B. Aspartate aminotransferase
   C. Creatine kinase
   D. Amylase
   E. Alkaline phosphatase

   Answer: E

5. In chronic liver failure there is a marked decrease of blood:
   A. Hemoglobin
   B. Bilirubin
   C. Immunoglobulin G
   D. Immunoglobulin M
   E. Albumin

   Answer: E

6. The most common malignant tumor of the liver is:
   A. Hepatocellular carcinoma
   B. Cholangiocellular carcinoma
   C. Kupffer cell sarcoma
   D. Carcinoid
   E. Metastatic tumor from another site

   Answer: E

7. Unconjugated hyperbilirubinemia is indicative of:
   A. Hemolytic jaundice
   B. Viral hepatitis
   C. Drug-induced hepatitis
   D. Hepatic tumor
   E. Extrahepatic biliary obstruction

   Answer: A

8. Unconjugated bilirubin circulates in the blood bound to:
   A. Immunoglobulin G (IgG)
   B. Albumin
   C. Haptoglobin
   D. Transferrin
   E. Ceruloplasmin

   Answer: B

9. Which of the following hepatitis viruses is a DNA virus with a protein envelope that contains several distinct antigens, such as surface antigen?
   A. HAV
   B. HBV
   C. HCV
   D. HDV
   E. HBV

   Answer: B

10. Which of the following hepatitis viruses is currently the most common cause of cirrhosis in the U.S.?
    A. HAV
    B. HBV
    C. HCV
    D. HDV
    E. HEV

    Answer: C

11. Overall the most common cause of cirrhosis in the U.S. is:
    A. Viral infection
    B. Alcohol abuse
    C. Drug abuse
    D. Immune hepatitis
    E. Extrahepatic obstruction

    Answer: B

12. In cirrhosis the surface of the liver is:
    A. Smooth and shiny
    B. Smooth but fatty
    C. Dark brown and rough
    D. Nodular
    E. Covered with fibrin or pus

    Answer: D

13. Complications of cirrhosis include all the following except:
    A. Ascites
    B. Splenomegaly
    C. Esophageal varices
    D. Hypoalbuminemia
    E. Hypogammaglobulinemia

    Answer: E

14. Accumulation of fluid in the abdominal cavity in patients with cirrhosis is associated with hypersecretion of which hormone?
    A. Insulin
    B. Glucagon
    C. Corticosteroids
    D. Aldosterone
    E. Androgen

    Answer: D

15. Which aspect of cirrhosis accounts for the development of esophageal varices?
    A. Portal hypertension
    B. Decreased level of fibrinogen in blood
    C. Retention of sodium
    D. Low osmolality of the plasma
    E. Hypersplenism

    Answer: A

16. In hemochromatosis the liver contains increased amounts of:
    A. Copper
    B. Zinc
    C. Iron
    D. Selenium
    E. Nickel

    Answer: C

17. In Wilson's disease the serum contains decreased amounts of:
    A. Hemosiderin
    B. Transferrin
    C. Ferritin
    D. Ceruloplasmin
    E. Haptoglobin

    Answer: D

18. Which of the following is the most common cause of cirrhosis in childhood?
    A. Hepatitis A virus infection
    B. Hepatitis D virus infection
    C. Hemosiderosis
    D. Alpha-1-antitrypsin deficiency
    E. Wilson's disease

    Answer: D

19. Which immunologic finding is most typical of primary biliary cirrhosis?
    A. Antinuclear antibodies
    B. Antismooth muscle antibodies
    C. Antimitochondrial antibodies
    D. Antimicrosomal antibodies
    E. Antinucleolar antibodies

    Answer: C

20. Primary sclerosing cholangitis affects primarily:
    A. Intercellular bile ductules along the liver cell plates
    B. Small intrahepatic bile ductules
    C. Small intrahepatic bile ducts
    D. Extrahepatic bile ducts
    E. Gallbladder

    Answer: D

21. In the preantibiotic era the most common cause of pylephlebitic abscesses of the liver was:
    A. Peptic ulcer
    B. Crohn's disease
    C. Ulcerative colitis
    D. Acute appendicitis
    E. Intestinal tuberculosis

    Answer: D

22. Yellow cholesterol gallstones are typically found in association with:
    A. Hemochromatosis
    B. Viral hepatitis
    C. Sickle cell anemia
    D. Chronic autoimmune hemolytic anemia
    E. Obesity

    Answer: E

23. Which of the following is a good serologic marker of hepatocellular carcinoma?
    A. Bilirubin
    B. Human chorionic gonadotropin
    C. Alpha fetoprotein (AFP)
    D. Alpha-1-antitrypsin (AAT)
    E. Alkaline phosphatase

    Answer: C

24. Gallbladder carcinoma is:
    A. More common in females than males
    B. More often squamous than adenocarcinoma
    C. More often invading the intestine than the liver
    D. More common in young people than old
    E. More often accompanied by jaundice than carcinoma of the common bile duct

    Answer: A

Clinicopathologic Review

Chapter 11—The Liver and Biliary Tract

Symptoms/Findings	Questions	Answers
A 30-year-old man became jaundiced 1 day after receiving a blood transfusion.	What type of hyperbilirubinemia is he likely to have?	Hemolysis leads to jaundice, which is primarily attributable to an excess of unconjugated bilirubin released from the RBCs.
A 20-year-old woman became jaundiced 3 weeks after vacationing in Mexico. She had no other symptoms.	What could be the cause of the jaundice?	In view of the history of travel to a tropical country, an infection should be suspected. Hepatitis A virus (HAV) infection may be acquired from contaminated food, and it is a well-known risk of travel abroad. The short incubation period and the mild disease favor the diagnosis of HAV infection. The diagnosis could be confirmed by demonstrating antibodies to HAV in the patient's serum.
The recipient of a heart transplant became jaundiced 8 weeks after the operation.	What could be the cause of jaundice in this patient?	Heart transplantation and other major operations require blood transfusion. Persons receiving blood transfusion can become infected with HBV or HCV if the blood has not been screened for these two viruses. Blood from donors who are serologically positive for HBV or HCV is not used for transfusion. Nevertheless, a small number of blood transfusions will result in hepatitis caused by a virus distinct from hepatitis viruses A, B, C, D, or E. The nature of these viruses has not yet been elucidated.

Copyright © 2000 by W.B. Saunders Company.   All rights reserved.

Symptoms/Findings *(con't)*	Question *(con't)*	Answer *(con't)*
A chronic alcoholic developed high fever, nausea, and vomiting, accompanied by jaundice, after a 3-day drinking binge.	What is the cause of this acute hepatitis?	Alcoholics are prone to infections that may be associated with fever secondary to pneumonia, upper respiratory infection, or some other inflammation. However, if an alcoholic develops fever and jaundice, especially after a prolonged drinking binge, one should consider the diagnosis of alcoholic hepatitis.
A chronic alcoholic presented with a protruding abdomen. Fluid was demonstrated in the abdominal cavity.	What is the cause of this ascites?	Ascites develops in alcoholics who have cirrhosis as a result of portal hypertension and hypoproteinemia and renal retention of sodium and fluids.
Ascites developed in a man with brown pigmentation of the skin, diabetes, and heart failure.	Which disease produces all of these symptoms?	Ascites (presumably secondary to cirrhosis), diabetes, heart disease, and skin pigmentation are typical features of hemochromatosis. This disease is characterized by deposits of hemosiderin in various organs. The iron in these deposits damages tissues and causes the functional defects that produce the typical symptoms described here.
A 40-year-old woman with mild jaundice noticed skin lesions in the form of small yellow plaques on her face, especially around the eyes.	What are these lesions?	This woman probably has xanthomas, which are yellow skin plaques or nodules composed of macrophages laden with lipid. Xanthomas are a common complication of hyperlipidemia that develops in primary biliary cirrhosis.
A 40-year-old man who had recently returned from Africa presented with diarrhea, painful enlargement of the liver, and fever.	What is the likely cause of his liver symptoms?	In a patient with a history of travel to the tropics and subsequent diarrhea, painful enlargement of the liver could represent abscesses that have developed as a complication of a tropical intestinal infection. Amebic infection should be suspected and appropriate treatment implemented.

Symptoms/Findings *(con't)*	Question *(con't)*	Answer *(con't)*
An obese 45-year-old woman developed spasmodic pain in the upper right quadrant of the abdomen 1 hour after ingesting a fat-laden meal.	What is the correct diagnosis?	Colic, or spasmodic pain in the upper right abdominal quadrant, is highly suggestive of biliary disease. Most often, biliary colic is caused by obstruction of the cystic duct with a gallstone. Symptoms typically occur following a heavy, fatty meal that stimulates contraction of the gallbladder and increased bile flow.
A 70-year-old woman, known to have gallstones, became jaundiced.	What is the probable cause of her jaundice?	Gallstones that enter the bile ducts may occlude the common bile ducts and cause jaundice. This obstructive jaundice may be attributable to other causes, however, so a diagnosis of biliary or pancreatic cancer should also be considered.
Sudden enlargement of the liver was noted in a 50-year-old man who was infected with hepatitis B virus during puberty and who developed signs of cirrhosis at the age of 40 years.	The differential diagnosis includes liver cancer. Which test should be ordered?	Alpha-fetoprotein (AFP) is the best serologic tumor marker for hepatocellular carcinoma, as serum levels are elevated in such cases. The diagnosis of liver cell cancer must, however, be confirmed by liver biopsy.

Chapter 12
The Pancreas

Instruction: Choose the one best answer.

1. The pancreas can be divided into several parts, the largest of which is the:
   A. Endocrine part
   B. Tail
   C. Head
   D. Body
   E. Accessory part

   Answer: C

2. Which of the following is a digestive enzyme secreted by the pancreas?
   A. Amylase
   B. Alkaline phosphatase
   C. Somatostatin
   D. Cholecystokinin
   E. Secretin

   Answer: A

3. Which component of the pancreatic juices acts as a buffer and neutralizes the acidity of the gastric juice?
   A. Amylase
   B. Lipase
   C. Peptidase
   D. Gastrin
   E. Bicarbonate

   Answer: E

4. Inadequate secretion of pancreatic digestive juices in chronic pancreatitis causes:
   A. Constipation
   B. Dilatation of the intestines
   C. Atrophy of the mucosa of the small intestine
   D. Malabsorption
   E. Jaundice

   Answer: D

5. Which of the following is an early sign of carcinoma of the head of pancreas?
   A. Hiccups
   B. Gastric regurgitation
   C. Jaundice
   D. Pain in the left upper abdominal quadrant
   E. Ascites

   Answer: C

6. Which of the following tumors has the highest incidence in 60–80-year-old American males?
   A. Insulinoma
   B. Somatostatinoma
   C. Gastrinoma
   D. Adenocarcinoma of the head of pancreas
   E. Adenocarcinoma of the papilla of Vater

   Answer: D

7. Which is the most important and most abundant hormone secreted by the pancreas?
   A. Insulin
   B. Glucagon
   C. Somatostatin
   D. Gastrin
   E. Cholecystokinin

   Answer: A

8. Acute pancreatitis can be induced experimentally by all the following except:
   A. Cholecystectomy
   B. Obstruction of the main pancreatic duct
   C. Mechanical disruption of the pancreatic acinar cells
   D. Drugs that injure pancreatic acinar cells
   E. Injection of bile into the main pancreatic duct

   Answer: A

9. Fat necrosis typically found in and around pancreas in acute pancreatitis is caused by a release of:
   A. Amylase
   B. Lipase
   C. Peptidase
   D. Pepsin
   E. Cholecystokinin

   Answer: B

10. Which of the following is a late complication of acute pancreatitis?
    A. Diverticulosis
    B. Amyloidosis
    C. Pseudocysts
    D. Carcinoma of the ducts of pancreas
    E. Zollinger-Ellison syndrome

    Answer: C

11. Typical pathologic findings in the pancreas affected by acute pancreatitis include all the following except:
    A. Edema of the head of pancreas
    B. Hemorrhage into the peripancreatic tissue
    C. Necrosis of peripancreatic fat tissue
    D. Foci of saponification around the pancreas
    E. Bacterial peritonitis

    Answer: E

12. Chronic pancreatitis is:
    A. More common than acute pancreatitis
    B. More common in males than females
    C. Associated with higher mortality than acute pancreatitis
    D. Associated with higher levels of amylase in blood than acute pancreatitis
    E. More common in children than in adults

    Answer: B

13. By x-ray the patients with chronic pancreatitis typically show:
    A. Edema of the head of pancreas
    B. Swelling of the tail of pancreas
    C. Distention of the papilla of Vater
    D. Calcifications of the pancreas
    E. Loss of endocrine cells from the pancreas

    Answer: D

14. The most prominent histologic feature of chronic pancreatitis is:
    A. Metaplasia
    B. Hyperplasia
    C. Fibrosis
    D. Ongoing necrosis
    E. Apoptosis

    Answer: C

15. Functionally most pancreatic carcinomas are characterized by:
    A. Hyperinsulinism
    B. Excess of glucagon
    C. Hypergastrinemia
    D. Excess of amylase
    E. No hormonal symptoms

    Answer: E

16. Histologically most carcinomas of the pancreas are classified as:
    A. Adenocarcinoma
    B. Oat cell carcinoma
    C. Squamous cell carcinoma
    D. Transitional cell carcinoma
    E. Acinic cell carcinoma

    Answer: A

17. Which of the following diagnostic approaches is most reliable for visualizing the carcinoma of the pancreas?
    A. Plain abdominal film
    B. CT scanning
    C. Laparoscopy
    D. Gastroscopy
    E. Colonoscopy

    Answer: B

18. A small pancreatic benign tumor that caused hypoglycemia and syncope is most likely:
    A. Insulinoma
    B. Glucagonoma
    C. VIPoma
    D. Gastrinoma
    E. Somatostatinoma

    Answer: A

19. Which of the following is most typical of diabetes mellitus?
    A. Oliguria
    B. Anuria
    C. Polyuria
    D. Proteinuria
    E. Cylindruria

    Answer: C

20. Primary diabetes mellitus is:
    A. Caused by viral infection
    B. Immune mediated
    C. Multifactorial
    D. Typically a disease of childhood
    E. Caused by pancreatic tumors

    Answer: C

21. Which of the following is the most common form of diabetes mellitus?
    A. Insulin dependent diabetes
    B. Noninsulin dependent diabetes
    C. Gestational diabetes
    D. Autosomal dominant form of diabetes
    E. Autosomal recessive form of diabetes

    Answer: B

22. Major biochemical abnormality typical of diabetes mellitus which can be detected by blood analysis is:
    A. Hypoglycemia
    B. Hyperglycemia
    C. Hyperamylasemia
    D. Hypoalbuminemia
    E. Hypercalcemia

    Answer: B

23. In early stages of insulin-dependent diabetes mellitus the typical pathologic finding is:
    A. Amyloidosis of islets of Langerhans
    B. Hyalinosis of islets of Langerhans
    C. Abscesses of islets of Langerhans
    D. Insulitis
    E. Hyperplasia of islets of Langerhans

    Answer: D

24. Typical renal complication of diabetes mellitus is:
    A. Glomerulonephritis
    B. Glomerulosclerosis
    C. Membranous nephropathy
    D. Tubular necrosis
    E. Hypertensive arterial changes

    Answer: B

Clinicopathologic Review

Chapter 12—The Pancreas

Symptoms/Findings	Question	Answer
Following two days of heavy drinking, a 40-year-old man developed upper abdominal pain.	You suspect acute pancreatitis. Which test should you order?	To document acute inflammation, one should order a white blood cell count (WBC). Leukocytosis (12,000–15,000 WBCs) is typically found. To prove that the inflammation involves the pancreas, one should measure serum levels of the pancreatic enzymes (amylase and lipase). An elevated concentration of amylase in the blood is evident during the first 24 hours of onset of the attack.
A 50-year-old alcoholic had a clinically documented attack of acute pancreatitis. A CT scan revealed a cystic mass in the pancreas.	What is this lesion?	In view of the history of acute pancreatitis, this is most likely a pseudocyst. In contrast to true cysts, which are lined with epithelium, pseudocysts do not have an epithelial lining. The wall of pseudocyst parenchyma is composed of granulation tissue and residual pancreatic parenchyma.
A chronic alcoholic had indigestion and bulky, foul-smelling, fatty stools.	What was the cause of steatorrhea?	Steatorrhea occurs as a result of malabsorption of fats from the intestinal lumen. Usually, it is a consequence of biliary or pancreatic disease. In chronic alcoholics, steatorrhea is often a sign of chronic pancreatitis.
A 70-year-old man with a history of weight loss, weakness, and nausea developed jaundice. Tests showed conjugated hyperbilirubinemia.	What is the cause of jaundice?	Conjugated hyperbilirubinemia suggests that this is obstructive jaundice, possibly caused by lesions, such as gallstones or tumors of the bile ducts or pancreas. In a patient with symptoms of general weakness, the cause is most likely carcinoma. Carcinoma of the head of the pancreas is a likely diagnosis. Other tumors, such as bile duct carcinoma, must be considered in the differential diagnosis.

Copyright © 2000 by W.B. Saunders Company. All rights reserved.

Symptoms/Findings *(con't)*	Question *(con't)*	Answer *(con't)*
A 20-year-old woman presented with a history of weight loss and urinary frequency. She reportedly ate a lot and was always thirsty.	What is the diagnosis?	Polyuria, polydipsia, and polyphagia associated with weight loss are common presenting signs of juvenile onset IDDM. Urine and serum glucose levels should be measured in this patient to determine whether she has hyperglycemia and glycosuria.
A 59-year-old diabetic had poor vision.	What could have caused this problem?	Diabetes is a common cause of pathologic changes in the eye. Visual problems could be a consequence of diabetic retinopathy, glaucoma, or cataracts.

Chapter 13
The Urinary Tract

Instruction: Match the numbered words or phrases with the most appropriate lettered item. Each lettered item can be used more than once.

- A. Bacterial infection
- B. Immunologic disorder
- C. Metabolic disorder
- D. Circulatory disorder
- E. Congenital/developmental disorder

1. Poststreptococcal glomerulonephritis
2. Acute pyelonephritis
3. Diabetic glomerulosclerosis
4. Prerenal renal failure
5. Dysuria
6. Polycystic kidney disease
7. Cystic renal dysplasia
8. Nephritic syndrome
9. Membranous nephropathy
10. Crescentic glomerulonephritis
11. Uric acid urinary stones
12. Struvite (ammonium magnesium sulfate) stones
13. Acute cystitis
14. Renocortical necrosis induced by shock
15. Hypertension due to renal artery stenosis

Answers: 1. B, 2. A, 3. C, 4. D, 5. A, 6. E, 7. E, 8. B, 9. B, 10. B, 11. C, 12. A, 13. A, 14. D, 15. D

Instruction: Match the numbered words or phrases with the most appropriate lettered item. Each lettered item can be used more than once.

- A. Pyuria
- B. Polyuria
- C. Hematuria
- D. Oliguria
- E. Glucosuria

16. Decreased daily output of urine
17. Blood in urine
18. Increased urine production
19. Excretion of sugar in urine
20. Pus in urine

Answers: 16. D, 17. C, 18. B, 19. E, 20. A

Instruction: Choose the one best answer.

21. Mercury poisoning affects mostly the:
    - A. Glomeruli
    - B. Proximal renal tubules
    - C. Distal renal tubules
    - D. Collecting ducts
    - E. Ureter

    Answer: B

22. All the following are features of acute glomerulonephritis except:
    A. Proteinuria
    B. Hematuria
    C. Polyuria
    D. Hypertension
    E. Edema

    Answer: C

23. All the following findings are typical of membranous nephropathy except:
    A. Proteinuria
    B. Pyuria
    C. Hypoalbuminemia
    D. Edema
    E. Deposits of immunoglobulin G in the glomeruli

    Answer: B

24. Which of the following is the most common cause of nephrotic syndrome in children?
    A. Membranous nephropathy
    B. Lipoid nephrosis
    C. Berger's disease (IgA nephropathy)
    D. Crescentic glomerulonephritis
    E. Poststreptococcal glomerulonephritis

    Answer: B

25. All the following are renal complications of diabetes except:
    A. Diffuse glomerulosclerosis
    B. Nodular glomerulosclerosis (Kimmelstiel-Wilson disease)
    C. Arteriolar hyalinosis
    D. Papillary necrosis
    E. Crescentic glomerulonephritis

    Answer: E

26. The most common urinary stones are composed of:
    A. Calcium phosphate
    B. Magnesium ammonium sulfate
    C. Uric acid
    D. Cystine
    E. Xanthine

    Answer: A

27. Acute "honeymoon" cystitis is caused by:
    A. Viruses
    B. Bacteria
    C. Parasites
    D. Fungi
    E. Mechanical irritation

    Answer: B

28. Hypertension of chronic kidney disease is medicated by:
    A. Erythropoietin
    B. Antidiuretic hormone
    C. Renin
    D. Calcitonin
    E. Adrenalin

    Answer: C

29. The most common malignant tumor of the urinary tract is:
    A. Renal cell carcinoma
    B. Wilms' tumor
    C. Carcinoma of renal pelvis
    D. Carcinoma of the ureter
    E. Carcinoma of the urinary bladder

    Answer: E

30. A solid renal tumor of a 4-year-old child was histologically composed ot immature cells reminiscent of fetal tubules. This tumor represents a(n):
    A. Renal cell adenoma
    B. Renal cell carcinoma
    C. Wilms' tumor
    D. Interstitial cell fibroma
    E. Teratoma

    Answer: C

31. Carcinoma of the urinary bladder is most often histologically classified as:
    A. Squamous cell carcinoma
    B. Adenocarcinoma
    C. Oat cell carcinoma
    D. Transitional cell carcinoma
    E. Seminoma

    Answer: D

Clinicopathologic Review
Chapter 13—The Urinary Tract

Symptoms/Findings	Question	Answer
The mother of a 3-month-old child palpated a mass on the left side of the child's abdomen.	What is this mass?	The three most common causes of abdominal masses in infants are multicystic renal dysplasia, Wilms' tumor, and neuroblastoma of the adrenals. Most likely, this mass is a developmentally abnormal kidney (i.e., multicystic renal dysplasia), but it could be a tumor as well.
A 40-year-old man has end-stage kidney failure and bilaterally enlarged kidneys.	What is the diagnosis?	Most patients with end-stage kidney disease have small kidneys, except when the renal failure is caused by autosomal dominant polycystic kidney disease (ADPKD). Although ADPKD is a congenital disease, symptoms of end-stage renal failure usually develop in the fourth decade of the patient's life.
A 4-year-old child developed puffiness around the eyes and became chronically sleepy 2 weeks after an episode of "strep-throat." The mother noted that the child's urine was dark brown and was being excreted in small amounts.	What is the probable diagnosis?	Edema, hematuria (accounting for the brown urine), and oliguria that develop 2 weeks after a streptococcal infection suggest the diagnosis of acute postinfectious glomerulonephritis. The child is somnolent, which could be attributable to brain edema caused by hypoalbuminemia or hypertension, which is typically found in such cases.
A 40-year-old man noticed generalized swelling, most prominently in his face and lower extremities. His physician discovered proteinuria and hypoalbuminemia.	What is the likely cause of edema in this case?	Generalized edema, proteinuria, and hypoalbuminemia are signs of nephrotic syndrome. In an adult, nephrotic syndrome is most often caused by membranous nephropathy. The diagnosis is confirmed by renal biopsy.

Symptoms/Findings (con't)	Question (con't)	Answer (con't)
A 40-year-old man noticed brown-red urine and, over a period of 6 days, stopped urinating altogether.	What is the probable diagnosis?	This man had acute oliguria that evolved into complete anuria. Without additional studies, it is not possible to determine the basis for his acute renal failure. Assuming that the disease is of glomerular origin because the renal failure was preceded by hematuria, one could speculate that the underlying disease is crescentic glomerulonephritis.
A diabetic patient developed sudden crampy pain radiating to the left back.	What could cause this pain?	Spasmodic pain radiating into the back is typical of renal colic, which is usually caused by obstruction of the ureter. In a diabetic, this may be attributable to papillary necrosis (i.e., sloughing off of the renal medullary papillae, which then float into the ureter, causing obstruction).
A 50-year-old man who underwent a routine medical checkup was found to have blood in his urine. X-ray studies revealed a renal mass on the left side.	What is the cause of his hematuria?	Hematuria associated with a renal mass in a 50-year-old man is highly suggestive of renal cell carcinoma. This man should have a nephrectomy.
A 20-year-old woman complained of pain during urination. She also noticed blood in her urine.	What is the most likely diagnosis?	Dysuria and hematuria are most often caused by cystitis. Urinary infections are common in young, sexually active adults, and are more common in women than in men.
A 60-year-old man noticed blood in the urine.	What should the work-up include?	The bleeding could be caused by cystitis or a tumor. The physician should send the urine for cytologic examination to determine whether there are tumor cells in the urine. A cystoscopy might also be performed to determine whether the urinary bladder contains tumors or stones, or whether it is only inflamed (cystitis). Cystitis in this age group could be secondary to prostatic hyperplasia.

Chapter 14
The Male Reproductive System

Instruction: Match the numbered words or phrases with the most appropriate lettered item. Each lettered item can be used more than once.

    A. Testis
    B. Epididymis
    C. Seminal vesicles
    D. Prostate
    E. Penis

1. Syphilitic chancre

2. Obstruction of sperm flow caused by sexually transmitted diseases

3. Orchitis

4. Seminoma

5. The site of most common carcinoma of old patients

6. The site of most common malignancy of male genital system in the 25–45 age group

7. Leydig cell tumor

8. Balanitis

9. Sertoli cell tumor

10. Yolk sac carcinoma

11. Nonseminomatous germ cell tumor

12. Benign nodular hyperplasia

    Answers: 1. E, 2. B, 3. A, 4. A, 5. D, 6. A, 7. A, 8. E, 9. A, 10. A, 11. A, 12. D

Instruction: Choose the one best answer.

13. All the following statements about infertility are true except:
    A. One in six couples in the U.S. is infertile.
    B. Infertility is as common among males as it is among females.
    C. Treatment of infertility costs society millions of dollars.
    D. Major advances have been made in the treatment of male infertility.
    E. Major advances have been made in the treatment of female infertility by in vitro fertilization.

    Answer: D

14. Most male genital infections are:
    A. Hematogenous
    B. Lymphogenous
    C. Sexually transmitted
    D. Caused by HIV
    E. Found before puberty

    Answer: C

15. An infertile man was found to have no scrotal testicles. Most likely diagnosis is:
    A. Klinefelter's syndrome
    B. Polyorchidism
    C. Cryptorchidism
    D. Orchitis
    E. Epididymoorchitis

    Answer: C

16. Typical manifestation of gonorrhea in males is:
    A. Orchitis
    B. Cystitis
    C. Inflammation of seminal vesicles
    D. Purulent urethritis
    E. Ulceration of the glans penis

    Answer: D

17. Genital herpes typically presents as:
    A. Painful prostatic enlargement
    B. Epididymitis
    C. Infertility
    D. Urethral papilloma
    E. Vesicles on the penis

    Answer: E

18. Which of the following is a typical feature of secondary syphilis?
    A. Penile ulcer
    B. Chancre on the prepuce
    C. Condyloma latum
    D. Aortic aneurysm
    E. Tabes dorsalis

    Answer: C

19. Most of the testicular tumors originate from:
    A. Germ cells
    B. Sertoli cells
    C. Leydig cells
    D. Stromal fibroblasts
    E. Tunica vaginalis testis

    Answer: A

20. Which of the following is a tumor marker of nonseminomatous germ cell tumors?
    A. Alkaline phosphatase
    B. Acid phosphatase
    C. Albumin
    D. Alpha fetoprotein
    E. Alpha antitrypsin

    Answer: D

21. Which of the following testicular tumors may cause premature puberty?
    A. Seminoma
    B. Yolk sac carcinoma
    C. Teratoma
    D. Leydig cell tumor
    E. Sertoli cell tumor

    Answer: D

22. The most common cause of prostatic enlargement in 60–70-year-old men is:
    A. Prostatitis
    B. Urethral obstruction
    C. Benign prostatic hyperplasia
    D. Prostatic adenoma
    E. Prostatic carcinoma

    Answer: C

23. Most carcinomas of the prostate:
    A. Present with symptoms of cystitis
    B. Present early in their course with urinary obstruction
    C. Invade early into the urethra
    D. Occur in the peripheral part (posterior lobe) of the prostate
    E. Tend to secrete androgens

    Answer: D

24. Invasive carcinoma of the prostate:
    A. Occurs mostly in old age
    B. Occurs more often in castrated men
    C. Is caused by HPV
    D. Is related to HIV infection
    E. Is a squamous cell carcinoma

    Answer: A

25. All the following are typical complications of prostatic enlargement except:
    A. Cystitis
    B. Urinary retention
    C. Hydroureters
    D. Hydronephrosis
    E. Glomerulonephritis

    Answer: E

26. Elevation of serum alkaline phosphatase in a patient with an enlarged prostate indicates that this man has:
    A. Prostatitis
    B. Benign prostatic hyperplasia
    C. Carcinoma in situ of the prostate
    D. Invasive carcinoma of the prostate that has spread to the urinary bladder
    E. Carcinoma of the prostate that has metastasized to the bone

    Answer: E

Clinicopathologic Review

Chapter 14—The Male Reproductive System

Symptoms/Findings	Question	Answer
A 3-month-old boy has a testis that is not palpable.	What is the diagnosis?	In approximately 4% of boys younger than 1 year of age, the testes are retractile and are found in the inguinal canal, rather than in the normal scrotal position. If the inguinal canal does not close by 1 year of age, the condition is considered to be a sign of cryptorchidism. Orchiopexy, or surgical positioning of the testis in the scrotum, should be performed.
In the same patient described above, the testis is still in the inguinal canal at 1 year of age.	Why should an orchiopexy be performed?	A cryptorchid testis, if left in an ectopic site, does not form sperm, and this could contribute to infertility. Furthermore, patients with undescended testes have a 10-fold greater risk for developing cancer than those with normally positioned testes.
Pain and induration developed in the epididymis of a promiscuous 20-year-old man.	What is the probable diagnosis and the cause of this condition?	This patient probably has epididymitis, or even epididymo-orchitis. Most likely, it is caused by a sexually transmitted pathogen, such as *Neisseria gonorrhoeae*, Chlamydia, or Mycoplasma. However, it could also be caused by an ascending infection from the urethra involving a uropathogen, such as *Escherichia coli*.
Small blisters were noticed on the glans penis in a 30-year-old man.	What is the most likely diagnosis?	Vesicles filled with clear fluid are typical signs of genital herpes.
A 20-year-old man noted a yellow urethral discharge 3 days after having casual sexual relations.	What is the likely diagnosis?	A purulent urethral discharge ("drip") most likely indicates gonorrhea. Treatment with penicillin will resolve the problem within days, usually without any residual symptoms or complications.

Symptoms/Findings *(con't)*	Question *(con't)*	Answer *(con't)*
A 60-year-old man complained of urgency and dribbling on urination.	What tests should be performed to establish the diagnosis?	In older men, urinary symptoms are most often related to prostatic enlargement. A rectal examination should be performed to determine whether the prostate is enlarged and painful. If it is painful, there is a good chance that it is inflamed. A urine culture should also be done to determine whether there is a superimposed infection. If urethritis or cystitis is confirmed, antibiotics should be administered. If the symptoms persist, a urologic examination, including cystoscopy, should be performed.
A testicular nodule was noticed by the patient on self-examination.	What is the appropriate work-up for this nodule?	If the testis contains a nodule, and especially if there is no evidence of inflammation, such as pain, swelling, or redness, the lesion should be surgically explored. If it proves to be a tumor, the tumor should be examined histologically and appropriate therapy prescribed.
A 35-year-old man with testicular cancer had a positive urine pregnancy test.	Does this test result mean that he is pregnant?	No! Men cannot be pregnant. However, positive results may be obtained from serologic or urinary hCG (pregnancy) testing in some patients with hCG-secreting testicular tumors. In all likelihood, this tumor is a NSGCT.

Symptoms/Findings *(con't)*	Question *(con't)*	Answer *(con't)*
Elevated serum levels of prostate specific antigen (PSA) and prostatic acid phosphatase (PAP) were detected in a 60-year-old man.	What is the significance of these findings?	PSA and PAP are markers of prostatic carcinoma. However, PAP and PSA are also produced and released by normal prostatic cells, and some of these substances may reach the blood of men with benign prostatic hyperplasia (BPH) and even of those with normal prostates. Thus, elevated PSA and PAP, without any evidence of prostatic cancer, should be interpreted cautiously. The patient should undergo ultrasonography, and multiple prostatic biopsies should be performed to exclude or confirm the diagnosis of cancer.
A 70-year-old man with sclerosis of the lumbar vertebrae had a rock-hard prostate on palpation.	Which serum enzyme tests would be expected to yield positive results?	Assuming (with considerable certainty) that this man has prostatic cancer with osteoblastic bone metastasis, one could predict that both the serum acid and alkaline phosphatase levels would be elevated. Acid phosphatase is produced by prostatic carcinoma cells, whereas alkaline phosphatase is released from osteoblasts forming the desmoplastic bone response to cancer.

Chapter 15
The Female Reproductive System

Instruction: Choose the one best answer.

1. Which of the following is part of the external female genitalia?
   A. Vagina
   B. Vulva
   C. Cervix
   D. Endometrium
   E. Fallopian tube

   Answer: B

2. All of the following infections of the female genital system are acquired by an ascending route except:
   A. Gonorrhea
   B. Syphilis
   C. Tuberculosis
   D. Chlamydial salpingitis
   E. Human papillomavirus infection

   Answer: C

3. Inflammation of the fallopian tubes is called:
   A. Cervicitis
   B. Endometritis
   C. Salpingitis
   D. Oophoritis
   E. Vulvovaginitis

   Answer: C

4. Which of the following is a protozoal cause of vaginitis?
   A. Gardnerella vaginalis
   B. Neisseria gonorrhoeae
   C. Treponema pallidum
   D. Trichomonas vaginalis
   E. Candida albicans

   Answer: D

5. Condyloma acuminatum is caused by:
   A. Herpes simplex virus type I
   B. Herpes simplex virus type II
   C. Human papillomavirus
   D. Chlamydia trachomatis
   E. Treponema pallidum

   Answer: C

6. Endometrial hyperplasia is typically a result of prolonged exposure to:
   A. Vitamin A
   B. Vitamin D
   C. Thyroid hormones
   D. Estrogen
   E. Progesterone

   Answer: D

7. The most common malignant neoplasm of female genital organs in the U.S. is carcinoma of the:
   A. Ovaries
   B. Fallopian tubes
   C. Endometrium
   D. Cervix
   E. Vagina

   Answer: C

8. All of the following tumors are squamous cell carcinoma except:
   A. Carcinoma of the vulva
   B. Carcinoma of the vagina
   C. Carcinoma of the cervix
   D. Carcinoma of the endometrium
   E. Carcinoma of the labia majora

   Answer: D

9. More than 50 percent of all cases of cervical intraepithelial neoplasia (CIN) contain intranuclear inclusions of:
   A. Gardnerella vaginalis
   B. Herpes simplex virus type I
   C. Herpes simplex virus type II
   D. Human papillomavirus
   E. Treponema pallidum

   Answer: D

10. Vaginal "spotting" (mild bleeding) after intercourse is most often seen in women who have:
    A. Carcinoma of the vulva
    B. Carcinoma of the cervix
    C. Carcinoma of the ovary
    D. Uterine leiomyoma
    E. Carcinoma of the fallopian tube

    Answer: B

11. All of the following are used in the treatment of cervical intraepithelial neoplasia except:
    A. Conization of the cervix with a scalpel
    B. Laser ablation
    C. Cryotherapy
    D. Electrocautery
    E. Dilatation and curettage (D&C)

    Answer: E

12. Which of the following endocrine disorders is a recognized risk factor for endometrial carcinoma?
    A. Hyperthyroidism
    B. Hypothyroidism
    C. Hyperestrinism
    D. Hypoparathyroidism
    E. Hyperinsulinism

    Answer: C

13. Women with carcinoma of the endometrium are at an increased risk of developing carcinoma of the:
    A. Ovary
    B. Vulva
    C. Adrenals
    D. Liver
    E. Lung

    Answer: A

14. In addition to the stage of the tumor the most important prognostic factor for women with endometrial carcinoma is:
    A. Age
    B. Presence of endocrine risk factors
    C. Obesity
    D. Hypertension
    E. History of irregular menstrual periods

    Answer: A

15. Most tumors of the endometrium are:
    A. Benign
    B. Premalignant
    C. Composed of striated muscle cells
    D. Found in postmenopausal women
    E. Found in prepubertal girls

    Answer: B

16. The most important complication of endometriosis is:
    A. Vaginal bleeding
    B. Infertility
    C. Pelvic inflammatory disease
    D. Polycystic ovary syndrome (POS)
    E. Malignant transformation

    Answer: B

17. A cystic ovarian lesion filled with clear, straw-colored fluid, showing multiple peritoneal metastases, is most likely a:
    A. Mucinous cystadenoma
    B. Mucinous cystadenocarcinoma
    C. Serous cystadenoma
    D. Serous cystadenocarcinoma
    E. Sertoli-Leydig cell tumor

    Answer: D

18. A cystic tumor that is lined from inside by skin and contains teeth in its wall is best classified as a:
    A. Granulosa cell tumor
    B. Thecoma
    C. Sertoli-Leydig cell tumor
    D. Teratoma
    E. Pseudomyxoma peritonei

    Answer: D

19. Abnormality of the placenta characterized by deep penetration of the placental villi into the wall of the uterus is called:
    A. Multiple placentae
    B. Placenta previa
    C. Placenta accreta
    D. Dichorionic diamniotic placenta
    E. Monozygotic pregnancy

    Answer: C

20. Most spontaneous abortions are consequences of:
    A. Developmental anomalies of the fetus and/or placenta
    B. Internal infections
    C. Autoimmune disorders
    D. Lack of estrogen in the maternal organism
    E. Excess of progesterone during early pregnancy

    Answer: A

21. Choriocarcinoma of pregnancy originates from the:
    A. Ovary
    B. Fallopian tubes
    C. Endometrium
    D. Placental trophoblastic cells
    E. Fetal cells in the placenta

    Answer: D

22. Swelling and cystic transformation of the placental villi resembling a bunch of grapes are typical of:
    A. Choriocarcinoma
    B. Hydatidiform mole
    C. Placenta accreta
    D. Placenta previa
    E. Endometriosis

    Answer: B

23. Eclampsia is characterized by all the following except:
    A. Hypertension
    B. Cerebral seizures
    C. Edema
    D. Proteinuria
    E. Hematuria

    Answer: E

24. Pap smear is most appropriate for early detection of:
    A. Choriocarcinoma
    B. Carcinoma of the ovary
    C. Endometrial carcinoma
    D. Carcinoma of the cervix
    E. Leiomyoma

    Answer: D

Clinicopathologic Review

Chapter 15—The Female Reproductive System

Symptoms/Findings	Question	Answer
Several days after a 20-year-old woman had intercourse with a casual acquaintance, she developed pain on urination and massive vaginal discharge.	Does this indicate an infection?	The symptoms of urethritis (dysuria) and cervicovaginitis (vaginal discharge) are strongly indicative of infection, possibly acquired by sexual intercourse.
A 17-year-old woman did not have her normal menstruation on the 28th day of the cycle. On the 38th day, she submitted a urine sample for a pregnancy test, with negative results.	What is the most likely cause of missed menstruation?	Many younger women, as well as those who are nearing menopause, have irregular menstrual cycles or miss menstruation because of functional disturbances of the hypothalamic-pituitary-ovarian axis. Many factors, including nervousness, can cause anovulation. Anovulatory bleeding usually occurs 2 to 3 weeks after the missed menstruation.
A 30-year-old woman noted blood (spotting) after intercourse.	What should she do?	Blood in the vaginal secretions after intercourse is not normal. Examination with a gynecologic speculum should be performed to determine whether the bleeding is from minor, intercourse-related trauma or a vaginal or cervical lesion. Remember that many early cancers of the cervix can present with spotting. As these are not always visible, it is essential that a Pap smear be obtained.
A 35-year-old woman received a report from her gynecologist indicating that she had a human papillomavirus (HPV) infection.	What is the significance of HPV infection?	As there are several types of HPV, the consequences of such infection depend on the type of virus isolated. Some HPV infections are innocuous and/or cause minor lesions (condyloma acuminata or venereal warts). Others cause cervical lesions that have a tendency to progress to cancer. Such infections should be monitored carefully.

Copyright © 2000 by W.B. Saunders Company.   All rights reserved.

Symptoms/Findings *(con't)*	**Question** *(con't)*	**Answer** *(con't)*
A 35-year-old woman complained of heaviness in the abdomen and a frequent urge to urinate. Gynecologic examination revealed an enlarged, bulky uterus.	What is the probable diagnosis?	The most common uterine tumor in women of reproductive age is a leiomyoma. Such tumors typically cause "mass symptoms"—that is, they compress the pelvic organs and cause a feeling of abdominal heaviness. Hysterectomy may be indicated, especially if the woman does not want to have any more children. Malignant uterine tumors are rare in woman younger than 40 years of age.
A 28-year-old woman had vague lower abdominal pain that intensified at the time of menstruation.	What is the possible cause of this pain?	Many women have painful menstruations, the cause of which cannot readily be identified. However, it is also known that about 15% of women have endometriosis that also causes pain, especially when there is bleeding into these lesions. Endometriotic lesions are often multiple and can be best identified by laparoscopy. Oral contraceptives may be used to suppress the cyclic bleeding, and the pain may resolve. If not, other hormonal therapy may be indicated.
A postmenopausal 52-year-old woman who had cessation of menstruation suddenly noted a bloody vaginal discharge.	What should she do?	A vaginal discharge that contains blood deserves scrutiny, especially in postmenopausal women. A gynecologist should determine whether the bleeding is from a vaginal, cervical, or uterine lesion. To this end, an inspection with a speculum must be performed. A Pap smear should be obtained and an endometrial biopsy performed. Remember that endometrial cancer is common in postmenopausal women, but if diagnosed early, it can be treated successfully. Endometrial biopsy is the best and most reliable method for diagnosing endometrial cancer.

Symptoms/Findings *(con't)*	**Question** *(con't)*	**Answer** *(con't)*
A 70-year-old woman noted abdominal swelling. The doctor diagnosed ascites and requested a gynecologic consultation.	What findings would be expected on gynecologic examination?	Ascites, or fluid in the abdominal cavity, is not normal. It can be caused by liver or heart failure, but it may also be caused by a tumor, most notably, an ovarian tumor metastatic to the peritoneum. Ascites and abdominal distention are quite common presenting signs of ovarian malignant tumors. Remember that ovarian malignant tumors seed over the abdominal cavity and either secrete serous fluid or cause transudation of fluid from the circulation into the abdominal cavity. Malignant cells can be detected in the ascites fluid.
A 30-year-old woman stopped menstruating and developed chest hair.	What should she do?	She should consult a gynecologist. Amenorrhea (no menstruation) and mild virilization are symptoms of hormonal disturbances, usually involving an excess of androgens. An excess of androgen (assuming that she is not injecting androgen "for kicks") could be of ovarian or adrenal origin, and a detailed hormonal work-up is indicated. Hormone-secreting tumors should be considered in the differential diagnosis. The tumor could involve the ovary (Sertoli-Leydig cell tumor) or the adrenals. More often, mild virilization is the result of functional ovarian disorders, such as polycystic ovary syndrome (POS) or disturbances of the hypothalamic-pituitary-ovarian axis.

Symptoms/Findings *(con't)*	Question *(con't)*	Answer *(con't)*
A 20-year-old promiscuous woman missed her period and presented 2 months later with sharp lower abdominal pain.	What is the first diagnosis that should be considered?	In women of reproductive age, lower abdominal pain and missed menstruation strongly suggest the possibility of an ectopic pregnancy. Even though similar symptoms may be caused by appendicitis, ectopic pregnancy is the first diagnosis that should be excluded. This can be diagnosed relatively easily by performing a pelvic examination and a pregnancy test.
A pregnant woman who had no previous prenatal care presented to the emergency room 5 months after her last menstrual period complaining of spotting. An enlarged uterus, corresponding to a 7-month pregnancy, was noticed. No fetal movement was evident.	What is the most likely diagnosis?	A missed abortion (i.e., intrauterine death of the fetus) can cause some of these symptoms, such as lack of fetal sounds and movement, but is not associated with enlargement of the uterus. Thus, one should consider the diagnosis of hydatidiform mole. The diagnosis of mole is best established by ultrasonographic studies. In addition, serum levels of hCG are high in such cases.

Chapter 16
The Breast

Instruction: Match the numbered words or phrases with the most appropriate lettered item. Each lettered item can be used more than once.

- A. Acute mastitis
- B. Gynecomastia
- C. Fibrocystic change
- D. Fibroadenoma
- E. Infiltrating duct carcinoma

1. Caused by invasion of lactiferous ducts with bacteria

2. Hormonally-induced enlargement of one or both breasts in males

3. The most common benign tumor of the breast

4. The most common cause of bilateral nodularity of the breast in premenopausal women

5. Typically presents as an indurated mass, adherent to other breast tissues, or fixated to the skin

6. A round mobile breast mass in a 20-year-old woman

7. A 45-year-old woman complained of painful "fullness" of the breast that fluctuates during the normal menstrual cycle. The breasts appeared "beady" and sensitive on palpation.

8. Swollen and somewhat enlarged left breast in a man who had cirrhosis of the liver caused by chronic alcohol abuse

9. A breast mass was aspirated by fine needle biopsy. The cytologic smear contained clumps of atypical cells that had high nuclear cytoplasmic ratio and hyperchromatic irregular nuclei

10. A tumor composed of elongated ducts composed of regular cuboidal cells, surrounded by loose connective tissue stroma

11. A painful and warm breast mass in a woman three days after delivery

Answers: 1. A, 2. B, 3. D, 4. C, 5. E, 6. D, 7. C, 8. B, 9. E, 10. D, 11. A

Instruction: Choose the one best answer.

12. In contrast to nonfunctioning breasts, the breast of late pregnancy and postpartum period contains:
    A. Periareolar ducts
    B. Hyperplastic subareolar ducts
    C. More connective tissue stroma
    D. More epithelial buds
    E. Acini

    Answer: E

13. Breast secretes milk in response to hormonal stimulation with:
    A. Estrogen
    B. Progesterone
    C. Prolactin
    D. Oxytocin
    E. Aldosterone

    Answer: C

14. Approximately 75 percent of all the lymph draining from the breast flows into the:
    A. Axillary lymph nodes
    B. Internal mammary lymph nodes
    C. External mammary lymph nodes
    D. Substernal lymph nodes
    E. Cervical lymph nodes

    Answer: A

15. Acute mastitis is most often caused by:
    A. Staphylococcus
    B. *E. coli*
    C. Mycobacterium tuberculosis
    D. Herpes virus
    E. Toxoplasma gondii

    Answer: A

16. All the following are features of fibrocystic disease of the breast except:
    A. Fibrosis
    B. Cystic change
    C. Epithelial cell proliferation
    D. Adenosis
    E. Cystosarcoma

    Answer: E

17. If a woman has a family history of cancer; i.e., her mother and her sister had cancer of the breast, her chances of developing breast cancer are:
    A. The same as in any other woman
    B. Somewhat increased (1–2 times)
    C. Slightly increased (2–3 times)
    D. Significantly increased (5–6 times)
    E. Very high and she will inevitably develop breast cancer

    Answer: D

18. A woman who was diagnosed with a stage I breast cancer, with no metastases, underwent a lumpectomy. Her chances of surviving 5 years are:
    A. 0
    B. 10%
    C. 25%
    D. 50%
    E. 80%

    Answer: E

19. All the following are used successfully in the treatment of breast cancer except:
    A. Anti-estrogen drugs
    B. Cytotoxic drugs
    C. Surgery
    D. Radiation therapy
    E. Hypnosis

    Answer: E

20. Fine needle aspiration biopsy of breast masses has an accuracy of:
    A. 100%
    B. 95%
    C. 75%
    D. 50%
    E. 25%

    Answer: B

21. Which of the following is the most common histologic type of breast carcinoma?
    A. Medullary carcinoma
    B. Mucinous carcinoma
    C. Infiltrating duct carcinoma
    D. Lobular carcinoma
    E. Tubular carcinoma

    Answer: C

Clinicopathologic Review
Chapter 16—The Breast

Symptoms/Findings	Question	Answer
A 3-cm breast mass was found in a 20-year-old woman.	What is the most likely diagnosis?	The most common tumor in young women is fibroadenoma. This tumor presents as a well-circumscribed mass that is unattached to surrounding breast tissue.
Painful small nodules of the breast were noted in a 40-year-old woman.	What is the most likely diagnosis?	Painful, finely nodular breast masses are typical of fibrocystic disease. In most cases, the findings are so typical that no biopsy is indicated. However, if a mammogram reveals suspicious areas, or if firm nodules distinct from the remaining breast are palpated, a biopsy should be performed.
A 3-cm mass was palpated in the breast of a 45-year-old woman.	What is the most likely diagnosis?	Any breast lump in women older than 35 years of age deserves to be examined most carefully. If the lump is firm and is attached to the skin or the underlying muscle, it is most likely a carcinoma. A breast biopsy should be performed.
Calcification and a small 0.5-cm mass were seen on mammography in a 50-year-old woman.	What should be done?	Small calcifications and an area of density indicative of a mass are common early signs of carcinoma. Biopsy of the lesion should be performed as soon as possible, and if the biopsy reveals malignant cells, the lesions should be surgically removed.
A woman known to have breast cancer also had a fracture of the leg.	What is the most likely cause of the fracture?	It is well known that breast cancer tends to metastasize to the bones. These metastases can cause pathologic fractures. X-ray studies are indicated.

Copyright © 2000 by W.B. Saunders Company.   All rights reserved.

Symptoms/Findings *(con't)*	Question *(con't)*	Answer *(con't)*
A painful mass was detected in the breast of a lactating woman.	What is the diagnosis?	Lactating breasts are prone to infection. A mass that develops in a lactating woman thus may represent dilated breast ducts filled with milk. However, if the mass is painful, red and warm, it is most likely the result of mastitis. The milk should be evacuated, and if the signs of inflammation do not subside, antibiotics should be administered.
Enlargement of the left breast was noted in a 40-year-old male patient with an adrenal tumor.	What is the diagnosis?	Enlargement of the male breast is called gynecomastia. It may be bilateral or unilateral. Gynecomastia is usually caused by an excess of estrogens in the blood. In a patient with an adrenal tumor, the estrogens are probably derived from the tumor cells which, like the normal adrenal, may secrete steroid hormones, including estrogens.

Chapter 17
The Endocrine System

Instruction: Choose the one best answer.

1. All the following are endocrine glands except:
   A. Pituitary
   B. Thyroid
   C. Spleen
   D. Adrenals
   E. Parathyroids

   Answer: C

2. The effect of hormones released into blood circulation and carried to a distant effector organ is called:
   A. Neuroendocrine
   B. Endocrine
   C. Paracrine
   D. Merocrine
   E. Autocrine

   Answer: B

3. Which of the following endocrine organs is located intracranially inside the sella turcica?
   A. Pituitary
   B. Parathyroid
   C. Thyroid
   D. Adrenal
   E. Pancreas

   Answer: A

4. The destruction of hypothalamus will lead to atrophy of all the following endocrine glands except:
   A. Pituitary
   B. Parathyroid
   C. Thyroid
   D. Adrenals
   E. Ovaries

   Answer: B

5. Tumors of the pituitary may secrete any one of the following hormones except:
   A. Growth hormone
   B. Prolactin
   C. Follicle-stimulating hormone
   D. Thyroid-stimulating hormone
   E. Cortisol

   Answer: E

6. The posterior pituitary or neurohypophysis releases:
   A. Gonadotropins
   B. ACTH
   C. Antidiuretic hormone
   D. Thyrotropin
   E. Prolactin

   Answer: C

7. The C cells of the thyroid secrete:
   A. Thyroglobulin
   B. Thyroxin
   C. Triiodothyronine
   D. Calcitonin
   E. Thyroid-stimulating hormone

   Answer: D

8. Which of the following hormones regulates the homeostasis of potassium and sodium?
   A. Calcitonin
   B. Parathyroid hormone
   C. Androgen
   D. Aldosterone
   E. Glucagon

   Answer: D

9. Epinephrine is secreted by:
   A. Adrenal zona glomerulosa
   B. Adrenal zona fasciculata
   C. Adrenal zona reticularis
   D. Adrenal medullary cells
   E. Adrenal cortical adenomas

   Answer: D

10. Prolonged adrenal stimulation with ACTH results in:
    A. Adrenal medullary hyperplasia
    B. Adrenal cortical hyperplasia
    C. Adrenal adenoma formation
    D. Adrenal cortical atrophy
    E. Adrenal medullary atrophy

    Answer: B

11. Adrenal hypofunction (Addison's disease) may be caused by all except:
    A. Adrenal tuberculosis
    B. Bilateral primary adrenal carcinoma
    C. Metastases of breast carcinoma to the adrenals
    D. Autoimmune adrenalitis
    E. Adrenal cortical hyperplasia

    Answer: E

12. ACTH, which is normally produced by pituitary cells, can also be produced by cells of the:
    A. Brain tumor
    B. Adrenal tumor
    C. Carcinoma of the thyroid
    D. Small cell carcinoma of the lung
    E. Ovarian carcinoma

    Answer: D

13. Amenorrhea and galactorrhea are typically produced by tumors which are classified as:
    A. Pituitary carcinoma
    B. Somatostatinoma
    C. Glucagonoma
    D. Prolactinoma
    E. Corticotropic adenoma

    Answer: D

14. Acromegaly is typically produced by tumors of the:
    A. Pituitary
    B. Thyroid
    C. Parathyroid
    D. Adrenals
    E. Testis

    Answer: A

15. General weakness, cold intolerance, poor appetite, weight loss following a delivery are typical of:
    A. Cushing's syndrome
    B. Sheehan's syndrome
    C. Cushing's disease
    D. Adrenogenital syndrome
    E. Graves' disease

    Answer: B

16. Graves' disease is caused by a disorder best classified as:
    A. Benign tumor
    B. Malignant tumor
    C. Infection
    D. Autoimmune disease
    E. Hormonal insufficiency

    Answer: D

17. Exophthalmos is a feature of:
    A. Hypothyroidism
    B. Graves' disease
    C. Hashimoto's thyroiditis
    D. Congenital thyroid aplasia
    E. Iodine deficiency

    Answer: B

18. Thyroid enlargement is most often caused by:
    A. Graves' disease
    B. Papillary carcinoma
    C. Follicular carcinoma
    D. Medullary carcinoma
    E. Idiopathic goiter

    Answer: E

19. Which of the following is the most common thyroid tumor?
    A. Follicular adenoma
    B. Follicular carcinoma
    C. Anaplastic carcinoma
    D. Papillary carcinoma
    E. Medullary carcinoma

    Answer: A

20. The most common cause of hyperparathyroidism is:
    A. Pituitary adenoma
    B. Parathyroid adenoma
    C. Parathyroid hyperplasia
    D. Medullary carcinoma of the thyroid
    E. Multiple endocrine neoplasia syndrome

    Answer: B

21. Secondary hyperparathyroidism is typically caused by:
    A. Hypovitaminosis A
    B. Hypovitaminosis D
    C. Hypovitaminosis C
    D. Chronic renal disease
    E. Chronic liver disease

    Answer: D

22. Nephrocalcinosis is a typical complication of adenoma of the:
    A. Pituitary
    B. Parathyroid
    C. Thyroid
    D. Adrenals
    E. Testis

    Answer: B

23. Hypocalcemic tetany is most often secondary to:
    A. Neck surgery
    B. Autoimmune disease
    C. Infectious disease
    D. Benign tumors
    E. Hyperparathyroidism

    Answer: A

24. What is the color of adrenal adenoma typically found in Cushing's syndrome?
    A. White
    B. Red
    C. Blue
    D. Yellow
    E. Black

    Answer: D

25. The most common cause of Cushing's syndrome encountered in medical practice today is:
    A. Adenoma of the pituitary
    B. Adenoma of adrenal cortex
    C. Adenoma of adrenal medulla
    D. Carcinoma of adrenal cortex
    E. Exogenous steroids administered by physicians

    Answer: E

26. Secondary hyperaldosteronism is typically a complication of chronic:
    A. Adrenal disease
    B. Renal disease
    C. Diabetes
    D. Idiopathic hypertension
    E. Emphysema

    Answer: B

27. Addison's disease is treated with:
    A. Aspirin
    B. Antihypertensive drugs
    C. ACTH
    D. Prolactin
    E. Corticosteroids

    Answer: E

28. Neuroblastomas have peak incidence in which age group?
    A. 1–5 years
    B. 10–15 years
    C. 20–25 years
    D. 40–45 years
    E. 60–65 years

    Answer: A

29. The most important clinical finding in patients with pheochromocytomas is:
    A. Hyperglycemia
    B. Hypertension
    C. Hyperestrinism
    D. Hypocalcemia
    E. Polyuria

    Answer: B

Clinicopathologic Review

Chapter 17—The Endocrine System

Symptoms/Findings	Question	Answer
A 30-year-old woman who is not pregnant has not menstruated for 4 months and is producing milk from her breasts.	What is the diagnosis?	This syndrome is called galactorrhea-amenorrhea syndrome. Most likely, the syndrome is caused by a prolactin-secreting pituitary adenoma.
A 40-year-old man noticed enlargement of his feet (suddenly ill fitting shoes) and hands. He had a prominent lower jaw and noticed that his teeth were becoming separated from one another.	What could have caused these symptoms?	Enlargement of the feet, hands, and jaw is typical of acromegaly, which is caused by growth hormone-secreting tumors of the pituitary.
A 45-year-old woman presented with complaints of sweating a lot, feeling hot and being constantly tired. She had a fast pulse rate and also reported feeling constantly hungry. On examination she was found to have bulging eyes and an enlarged thyroid.	What is the diagnosis?	These symptoms could be explained by hypermetabolism, which is typical of hyperthyroidism. This woman's bulging eyes (proptosis), in combination with her thyroid enlargement and hypermetabolism, indicate that she has Graves' disease.
A 30-year-old woman noticed a "swelling" on the anterior side of her lower neck. She had no other symptoms.	What should she do?	This woman should see her physician, who will examine her to determine the nature of this neck mass. Assuming that the mass represents a thyroid mass, the physician must establish whether this is a solitary nodule or a goiter involving the entire lobe or even the entire thyroid. Most likely, the enlargement is caused by a hormonally inactive, multinodular goiter.
A 35-year-old woman was diagnosed with papillary carcinoma localized to one lobe of the thyroid.	What is the prognosis?	Papillary carcinoma of the thyroid has a very good prognosis, especially if diagnosed early and removed completely.

Symptoms/Findings *(con't)*	Question *(con't)*	Answer *(con't)*
A 50-year-old man with urinary stones was found to have elevated blood concentrations of parathyroid hormone (PTH).	What should be done next?	Elevated PTH blood concentrations are diagnostic of hyperparathyroidism. If the patient has normal kidneys, the disease is most likely caused by parathyroid hyperplasia or adenoma, which may be treated surgically.
A neonate developed spastic seizures soon after birth. Hypocalcemia was diagnosed on the basis of biochemic studies.	What could be the cause of this child's hypocalcemia?	Muscular spasms secondary to hypocalcemia in infants could be the first symptoms of hypoparathyroidism. In that age group, hypoparathyroidism is typically caused by agenesis of the parathyroid glands, which is associated with agenesis of the thymus. This disease is called DiGeorge's syndrome.
A 50-year-old man became extremely obese, with fat accumulating most markedly on his trunk. He had a red, rounded face and almost translucent thin skin that was prone to bruising.	What is the first question that should be posed to this man?	The symptoms and findings described suggest Cushing's syndrome or Cushing's disease. However, primary endogenous hypercortisolism is rare, in comparison with the incidence of drug-induced Cushing's syndrome. Thus, one should first establish whether this patient is receiving corticosteroids for some disease (e.g., rheumatoid arthritis or asthma). If exogenous steroids are excluded, the patient should be evaluated to determine whether he has a pituitary ACTH-secreting tumor or an adrenal tumor, or adrenal hyperplasia.
A 40-year-old man reported having sudden attacks of dizziness, blurred vision, and excruciating headaches. During these attacks, his blood pressure was 180/120 mm Hg.	What could cause these paroxysms of hypertension?	Pheochromocytoma, a tumor of the adrenal medulla which secretes epinephrine and norepinephrine, may cause sudden bouts of hypertension that correlate with a periodic release of these vasoactive amines into the circulation. Typically, such patients have increased amounts of catecholamines in urine.

Chapter 18
The Skin

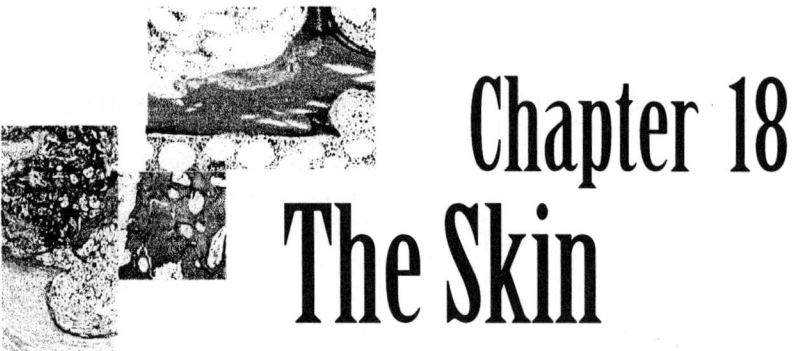

Instruction: Match the numbered words or phrases with the most appropriate lettered items. Each lettered item can be used more than once.

- A. Infectious disease
- B. Idiopathic disease
- C. Immune disease
- D. Neoplastic disease
- E. Disease caused by exogenous physical factors

1. Immersion foot
2. Frostbite
3. Sunburn
4. Impetigo
5. Folliculitis
6. Furuncle (boil)
7. Carbuncle
8. Dermatophytosis
9. Tinea corporis
10. Mycetoma
11. Verruca vulgaris
12. Acne
13. Eczema, exogenous
14. Seborrheic dermatitis
15. Psoriasis
16. Seborrheic keratosis
17. Superficial spreading melanoma
18. Kaposi's sarcoma
19. Mycosis fungoides
20. Urticaria pigmentosa

Answers: 1. E, 2. E, 3. E, 4. A, 5. A, 6. A, 7. A, 8. A, 9. A, 10. A, 11. A, 12. A, 13. C, 14. B, 15. B, 16. D, 17. D, 18. D, 19. D, 20. D

Instruction: Choose the one best answer.

21. Diabetes predisposes the skin to:
    A. Tumors
    B. Autoimmune diseases
    C. Infections
    D. Hyperplasia
    E. Hyperpigmentation

    Answer: C

22. Bullae may be caused by all the following except:
    A. Sunbathing
    B. Allergic reaction
    C. Poison ivy
    D. Porphyria
    E. Tumors

    Answer: E

23. Flat, slightly pigmented skin patch measuring 1 cm is best classified as a:
    A. Macule
    B. Papule
    C. Pustule
    D. Vesicle
    E. Bulla

    Answer: A

24. Which of the following tends to present as an ulcer?
    A. Psoriasis
    B. Eczema
    C. Syphilitic chancre
    D. Ichthyosis
    E. Albinism

    Answer: C

25. Prolonged suntanning causes:
    A. Ulcers
    B. Accelerated aging of the skin
    C. Furuncles
    D. Carbuncles
    E. Psoriasis

    Answer: B

26. Impetigo is typically caused by:
    A. Herpesvirus
    B. Human papillomavirus
    C. Streptococci
    D. Fungi
    E. Scabies

    Answer: C

27. Ringworm lesions are caused by:
    A. Worms
    B. Parasites
    C. Fungi
    D. Bacteria
    E. Viruses

    Answer: C

28. Measles present with:
    A. Maculopapular rash
    B. Vesicular eruption
    C. Bullous eruption
    D. Disseminated furunculosis
    E. Ulcerations

    Answer: A

29. The most common epithelial malignant tumor of the face is:
    A. Fibroma
    B. Basal cell carcinoma
    C. Squamous cell carcinoma
    D. Malignant melanoma
    E. Lymphoma

    Answer: B

30. Preinvasive carcinoma of the sun-exposed skin is called:
    A. Seborrheic keratosis
    B. Seborrheic dermatitis
    C. Actinic keratosis
    D. Basal cell carcinoma
    E. Mycosis fungoides

    Answer: C

31. Malignant melanoma may originate from:
    A. Seborrheic keratosis
    B. Basal cell carcinoma
    C. Lentigo
    D. Urticaria pigmentosa
    E. Mycosis fungoides

    Answer: C

32. Which of the following pigmented lesions has the highest propensity to progress to malignant melanoma?
    A. Ephelis
    B. Lentigo
    C. Dermal nevus
    D. Blue nevus
    E. Dysplastic nevus

    Answer: E

33. Which of the following neoplastic lesions originates in the dermis rather than epidermis?
    A. Basal cell carcinoma
    B. Squamous cell carcinoma
    C. Actinic keratosis
    D. Dermatofibroma
    E. Seborrheic keratosis

    Answer: D

Clinicopathologic Review

Chapter 18—The Skin

Symptoms/Findings	Question	Answer
An infant was born with very white skin, white hair, and red eyes.	What is the underlying defect?	Generalized lack of pigment is called albinism. The melanocytes do not produce melanin because of a genetic deficiency of melanin-synthesizing enzymes (e.g., tyrosinase deficiency).
Blisters formed on the skin of a woman who had been suntanning.	What is the mechanism of bullae formation?	The sunlight injury by infrared thermal rays causes epidermal cell necrosis and loosening of the intercellular junctions, which is accompanied by an influx of plasma into intercellular spaces and formation of bullae.
A vesicular rash erupted over the entire body of a 3-year-old.	What is the probable cause of the rash?	Systemic vesicular exanthem in a small child is most likely chickenpox. This viral disease has a limited course and heals within a week after the onset of eruption.
Numerous pus-containing pimples developed on the face of a 17-year-old.	Is this disease related to masturbation?	No. Pimples on the face of teenagers are typical of acne. The cause of acne is not fully understood, but it has nothing to do with masturbation, sexual abstinence, or diet, despite folkloric claims to the contrary.
Itchy, rough-surfaced, oozing lesions were noted on the skin of a 3-year-old child.	What is the diagnosis?	This is eczema. Note that eczema is not a single disease and it could have many causes. In childhood, the most common disease is atopic dermatitis, a disease of presumptive immune pathogenesis that runs in families.

Symptoms/Findings *(con't)*	Question *(con't)*	Answer *(con't)*
A 20-year-old man had pearly skin papules that were most prominent on the elbows and knees.	Is this a contagious disease?	No. Most likely, this is psoriasis, a multifocal disease with a predilection for easily traumatized extensor surfaces of the arms and legs. Psoriasis is related to an epidermal cell proliferation defect, and is not caused by infectious agents.
Blisters erupted on the abdominal skin of a women treated for tuberculosis.	Are the blisters caused by the bacilli of tuberculosis?	No. Most likely, the skin blisters represent an allergic reaction to a drug used to treat tuberculosis. Drug reactions may take many forms, such as rash, papules, or vesicles.
A small, 5-mm nodule with a central non-healing ulceration was noticed on the cheek of a 60-year-old man.	What should be done?	Patients with persistent skin lesions that change their appearance or do not heal should undergo biopsy. In the elderly, this lesion may represent a basal cell epithelioma. It should be removed completely to avoid recurrence.
A 70-year-old man presented with a 7-mm brown lesion that was slightly elevated in one part, and pale and depressed in the center. It had irregular margins.	Could this be a melanoma?	This pigmentary lesion should be removed and examined histologically. It is asymmetrical, has irregular borders, appears variegated in color, and is larger than 6 mm in diameter. It has all the "A-B-C-D" aspects of melanoma.

Chapter 19
Bones and Joints

Instruction: Choose the one best answer.

1. The extracellular organic matrix of bones is called:
   A. Osteon
   B. Osteoid
   C. Osteoblast
   D. Osteocyte
   E. Osteoclast

   Answer: B

2. The central ("midshaft") portion of long bones is called:
   A. Epiphysis
   B. Metaphysis
   C. Diaphysis
   D. Physis
   E. Anapophysis

   Answer: C

3. Which vitamin is essential for the formation of bones?
   A. Vitamin A
   B. Vitamin B_1
   C. Vitamin B_{12}
   D. Vitamin D
   E. Vitamin E

   Answer: D

4. Softening of bones due to excessive resorption of calcium salts from the extracellular bone matrix is called:
   A. Osteoporosis
   B. Osteomalacia
   C. Osteopetrosis
   D. Osteitis deformans
   E. Pellagra

   Answer: B

5. Rheumatoid arthritis is best classified as:
   A. Infectious disease
   B. Degenerative disease
   C. Inborn error of metabolism
   D. Autoimmune disease
   E. Neoplastic disease

   Answer: D

6. Which of the following diseases is an autosomal dominant cause of dwarfism?
   A. Achondroplasia
   B. Osteopetrosis
   C. Osteogenesis imperfecta
   D. Rickets
   E. Osteomalacia

   Answer: A

7. Osteogenesis imperfecta is an inborn error in the synthesis of:
   A. Collagen type I
   B. Collagen type II
   C. Collagen type III
   D. Phosphate crystals
   E. Basement membranes

   Answer: A

8. Osteomyelitis of long bones is most often caused by:
   A. Viruses
   B. Pyogenic bacteria
   C. Mycobacterium tuberculosis
   D. Fungi
   E. Parasites

   Answer: B

9. Aseptic necrosis of bones may be caused by all the following except:
   A. Sickle cell anemia
   B. Thrombotic occlusion of a nutrient artery
   C. Trauma
   D. Bacteria
   E. Drugs

   Answer: D

10. Which of the following diseases has the highest incidence among postmenopausal women?
    A. Osteoporosis
    B. Osteopetrosis
    C. Osteomalacia
    D. Achondroplasia
    E. Osteomyelitis

    Answer: A

11. The excess of which hormone causes osteoporosis?
    A. Androgens
    B. Estrogens
    C. Corticosteroids
    D. Prolactin
    E. Glucagon

    Answer: C

12. Osteoporosis is usually diagnosed by means of:
    A. Bone biopsy
    B. Electron microscopy
    C. X-ray
    D. Analysis of blood
    E. Analysis of joint fluid

    Answer: C

13. Bowlegs, craniotabes, and rachitic rosary in a growing child are signs of:
    A. Osteoporosis
    B. Osteopetrosis
    C. Vitamin B_1 deficiency
    D. Vitamin D deficiency
    E. Vitamin A deficiency

    Answer: D

14. The bone lesions in renal osteodystrophy are caused by an excess of:
    A. ACTH
    B. Thyroglobulin
    C. Parathyroid hormone
    D. Aldosterone
    E. Androgens

    Answer: C

15. If a long bone fracture has numerous lines and fragments it is called:
    A. Simple
    B. Greenstick
    C. Comminuted
    D. Complete
    E. Incomplete

    Answer: C

16. Benign bone tumor composed of cartilage cells is called:
    A. Osteoma
    B. Chondroma
    C. Fibroma
    D. Paget's disease
    E. Ewing's disease

    Answer: B

17. The most common primary malignant tumor of bones is called:
    A. Osteosarcoma
    B. Chondrosarcoma
    C. Paget's disease
    D. Ewing's disease
    E. Giant-cell tumor of bone

    Answer: A

18. Osteosarcomas most often arise in the bones of the:
    A. Skull
    B. Vertebra
    C. Fingers
    D. Toes
    E. Knee

    Answer: E

19. A tumor in a 15-year-old boy was diagnosed in the diaphysis of the tibia. On x-ray it had a sunburst appearance and histologically it was composed of a uniform population of small blue cells. This tumor is a(n):
    A. Osteosarcoma
    B. Chondrosarcoma
    C. Giant cell tumor
    D. Ewing's sarcoma
    E. Metastasis from a lung cancer

    Answer: D

20. Which joint disease is characterized by destruction and loss of cartilage sclerosis of subchondral bone, cyst formation, and osteophytes'?
    A. Osteoarthritis
    B. Osteomalacia
    C. Rheumatoid arthritis
    D. Gout
    E. Infectious arthritis

    Answer: A

21. The most common symptom of degenerative joint disease is:
    A. Fever
    B. Swelling
    C. Pain
    D. Ankylosis
    E. Crepitation

    Answer: C

22. In rheumatoid arthritis the synovium of joints is infiltrated with:
    A. Neutrophils
    B. Eosinophils
    C. Mast cells
    D. Basophils
    E. Plasma cells

    Answer: E

23. Patients with so-called seropositive rheumatoid arthritis have in their blood antibodies to:
    A. Viruses
    B. Their own immunoglobulins
    C. Smooth muscle cells
    D. Cartilage
    E. Synovial membrane

    Answer: B

24. Subcutaneous nodules composed of a central area of fibrinoid necrosis surrounded by macrophages and lymphocytes are typical of:
    A. Infectious arthritis
    B. Rheumatoid arthritis
    C. Osteoarthritis
    D. Gout
    E. Rickets

    Answer: B

25. Migratory arthritis caused by Borrelia burgdorferi is typical of:
    A. Rocky Mountain spotted fever
    B. Trench foot
    C. Lyme disease
    D. Legionnaire's disease
    E. Osteoarthritis

    Answer: C

Clinicopathologic Review

Chapter 19—Bones and Joints

Symptoms/Findings	Questions	Answers
A child experienced easy fatigability and on examination was found to have anemia. X-ray studies showed dense bones. A diagnosis of osteopetrosis was established.	Why is the child anemic?	In osteopetrosis, the bone replaces the hematopoietic bone marrow, causing anemia.
A 12-year-old girl with sickle cell anemia developed pain in the knee. The pain was associated with bouts of fever.	What is the cause of these symptoms?	Sickling crisis may occlude small blood vessels of the bone and cause aseptic necrosis, which typically presents with pain. Such necrotic bone may serve as a focus for infection. Bouts of fever suggest that osteomyelitis has developed.

Symptoms/Findings *(con't)*	Question *(con't)*	Answer *(con't)*
A 65-year-old woman fell in the kitchen and broke her leg.	Does this woman have osteoporosis?	One may break a bone at any age, and a bone fracture does not mean that the affected person has osteoporosis. However, if fracture occurs following a minor accident or trauma, if there are multiple fractures, and if the person is elderly, one should look for signs of osteoporosis.
A 14-year-old boy developed pain in his knee after a softball game. X-ray studies disclosed an expansive mass in the distal end of the femur.	What is the diagnosis?	The x-ray findings suggest that this boy has a primary bone tumor. In order to make the final diagnosis, a biopsy of the lesion should be performed. The age of the patient and the location of the lesion favor the diagnosis of osteosarcoma.
A 60-year-old woman broke her upper arm. The radiologist characterized this as a "pathological fracture" and reported that the bone contained a tumor.	What is the nature of this tumor?	The term "pathological fracture" is used to describe fractures that have an underlying cause and are not simply attributable to trauma. In this case, the fracture was caused by a tumor. In the elderly, most bone tumors represent metastases from a malignant lesion in an internal organ. A biopsy must, nevertheless, be performed to confirm the diagnosis.
A 40-year-old woman complained of "morning stiffness" and pain in her hands. The pain responded well to aspirin.	What is the diagnosis?	The most likely diagnosis is rheumatoid arthritis, which is a very common disease. The disease may present with a variety of symptoms, but typically, most patients complain of joint pain. A good response to aspirin also favors this diagnosis.

Chapter 20
Muscles

Instruction: Choose the one best answer.

1. The transmission of impulses from the nerve to the striated muscle at the neuromuscular junction is mediated by the release of:
   A. Adrenaline
   B. Acetylcholine
   C. Cholinesterase
   D. Norepinephrine
   E. Acetaldehyde

   Answer: B

2. Skeletal muscles are:
   A. Composed of either type I (slow) or type II (fast) fibers
   B. Composed of rapidly dividing cells
   C. Composed of nondividing cells that can be stimulated to enter mitosis by a variety of cytokines
   D. In close contact with nerves
   E. Major storage site of calcium and phosphate

   Answer: D

3. Spastic contraction of muscles known as tetany is caused by:
   A. Hypercalcemia
   B. Hypoparathyroidism
   C. Hyperthyroidism
   D. Hyponatremia
   E. Hypophosphatemia

   Answer: B

4. Botulism, a disease caused by a toxin from Clostridium botulinum, is marked by:
   A. Tetany
   B. Convulsions
   C. Paralysis of muscles
   D. Loss of sensation
   E. Hypercalcemia

   Answer: C

5. All the following are autoimmune diseases affecting the muscles except:
   A. Myasthenia gravis
   B. Rheumatoid arthritis
   C. Systemic lupus erythematosus
   D. Duchenne's muscular dystrophy
   E. Dermatomyositis

   Answer: D

6. Destruction of muscle fibers in polymyositis is characterized by a release of enzymes, the most specific for muscle disease of which is:
   A. Lactate dehydrogenase
   B. Acid phosphatase
   C. Alkaline phosphatase
   D. Creatine kinase
   E. Alanine aminotransferase

   Answer: D

7. Peripheral motor neurons are extensions of nerve cells which are typically located in the:
   A. Cortex of the brain
   B. Basal ganglia
   C. Pons
   D. Medulla oblongata
   E. Anterior horn of the spinal cord

   Answer: E

8. Which of the following is a typical "upper neuron injury"?
   A. Polymyositis
   B. Guillain-Barre syndrome
   C. Spinal cord injury in traffic accident
   D. Diabetic neuropathy
   E. Lead poisoning

   Answer: C

9. Following wallerian degeneration the nerve function is restored by the:
   A. Regeneration of dendrites from the perikaryon
   B. Regeneration of the axon from the peripheral parts of the transected nerve
   C. Regeneration of the axon from the proximal portion of the transected axon
   D. Loss of the perikaryon
   E. Loss of the Nissl substance

   Answer: C

10. First symptoms of myasthenia gravis among women appear most often in which age group?
    A   0–5 years
    B. 5–20 years
    C. 20–35 years
    D. 35–50 years
    E. Over 50 years

    Answer: C

11. Almost all patients with myasthenia gravis show:
    A. Signs of muscle degeneration
    B. Regrouping of type I and type II muscles
    C. Muscle atrophy
    D. Antibodies to acetylcholine
    E. Antibodies to acetylcholine receptor

    Answer: E

12. Patients with myasthenia gravis given edrophonium, an antagonist of cholinesterase, show:
    A. Aggravation of symptoms
    B. Complete paralysis
    C. Temporary improvement of muscle weakness
    D. Reduced levels of circulating antibodies
    E. Reduced calcium in blood

    Answer: C

13. A patient with myasthenia gravis was found to have an anterior mediastinal mass. This mass proved to be a tumor. Most likely it is a:
    A. Thyroid adenoma
    B. Parathyroid adenoma
    C. Neuroblastoma
    D. Smooth muscle cell tumor
    E. Thymoma

    Answer: E

14. Duchenne's muscular dystrophy is inherited as:
    A. Autosomal dominant trait
    B. Autosomal recessive trait
    C. Sex-linked recessive trait
    D. Sex-linked dominant trait
    E. Polygenic trait

    Answer: C

15. Symptoms of muscle weakness in Duchenne's dystrophy begin in:
    A. Preschool children
    B Elementary school children
    C. High school children
    D. College-level teenagers
    E. Adults

    Answer: A

16. Which of the following muscular dystrophies involves the same gene as Duchenne's dystrophy?
    A. Becker's dystrophy
    B. Limb-girdle dystrophy
    C. Facioscapulohumeral dystrophy
    D. Myotonic dystrophy
    E. Werdnig-Hoffmann disease

    Answer: A

17. Frontal baldness, testicular atrophy, and muscle spasm are typical of which autosomal dominant muscular dystrophy?
    A. Duchenne's
    B. Becker's
    C. Facioscapulohumeral
    D. Limb-girdle
    E. Myotonic

    Answer: E

18. Which is the most common cause of muscle weakness and/or paralysis in infants and children?
    A. Duchenne's dystrophy
    B. Becker's dystrophy
    C. Cerebral palsy
    D. Dermatomyositis
    E. Infectious myositis

    Answer: C

19. Which of the following viruses is the best-known cause of myositis?
    A. Herpesvirus type I
    B. Herpesvirus type II
    C. CMV
    D. Coxsackie virus
    E. Mumps virus

    Answer: D

20. Muscle inflammation characterized by infiltrates of lymphocytes and plasma cells is most typical of:
    A. Muscular dystrophy
    B. Muscular atrophy
    C. Trichinella spiralis infection
    D. Polymyositis
    E. Myasthenia gravis

    Answer: D

21. Malignant tumor of striated muscle is called:
    A. Leiomyosarcoma
    B. Rhabdomyosarcoma
    C. Liposarcoma
    D. Synovial sarcoma
    E. Malignant fibrous histiocytoma

    Answer: B

22. The most common histologic type of soft tissue sarcoma in adults is:
    A. Liposarcoma
    B. Malignant fibrous histiocytoma
    C. Rhabdomyosarcoma
    D. Leiomyosarcoma
    E. Synovial sarcoma

    Answer: B

Clinicopathologic Review

Chapter 20—Muscles

Symptoms/Findings	Question	Answer
A knife wound caused paralysis of the hand.	Can this be treated?	Yes. Transected nerves can be sutured together (i.e., surgically repaired). The axon will regenerate and reinnervate denervated muscles, thus reversing the paralysis.

Symptoms/Findings *(con't)*	Question *(con't)*	Answer *(con't)*
Muscle weakness was noticed in a diabetic patient.	What is the cause of this muscle weakness?	Diabetic patients suffer from muscle weakness that is multifactorial. Diabetic microangiopathy causes ischemic atrophy of muscle fibers. Diabetic neuropathy, marked by a loss of axonal branches, causes secondary neurogenic atrophy of muscle fibers. Metabolic abnormalities secondary to a deficiency of insulin also contribute to muscle weakness.
Myasthenia gravis was diagnosed in a 30-year-old woman.	What kind of antibodies does she have in circulation?	Essentially all patients with myasthenia gravis have antibodies to acetylcholine (ACh) receptor.
This same woman also had a mediastinal "shadow" on radiographic examination.	What does this shadow represent?	The shadow (i.e., a mass in the anterior mediastinum) is either a hyperplastic thymus or a thymoma. It should be resected. This could improve the patient's symptoms of myasthenia gravis.
Two sons of an asymptomatic woman had signs of muscular dystrophy by the age of 5 years. All daughters were normal.	What is the diagnosis?	The most likely diagnosis is Duchenne type muscular dystrophy, which affects only males and becomes evident in early childhood.
The creatine kinase (CK) was elevated above the normal level in the blood of a marathon runner.	Does this finding signify muscle disease?	The most likely cause of muscle enlargement in such patients is "pseudohypertrophy," caused by an accumulation of fat cells that replace the destroyed muscle cells.
The muscle around a deep wound became crepitant and appeared bubbly on palpation.	What could cause bubbles within the muscle?	No. CK blood levels are elevated in many muscle diseases marked by destruction of muscle cells, such as polymyositis and muscular dystrophy. However, trauma or overexertion may provoke rhabdomyolysis, which is also associated with CK elevations in blood.

Symptoms/Findings *(con't)*	Question *(con't)*	Answer *(con't)*
The shin muscle in a child with Duchenne type dystrophy appeared to be enlarged but soft and weak.	What is the reason for the enlargement of muscles in muscular dystrophy?	Bubbles in the muscle surrounding a wound could be the first sign of gas gangrene. Such Clostridial infections have high mortality and are best prevented by careful surgical cleansing of the wound and the surrounding necrotic tissues.
A skin rash developed over the face of a 12-year-old girl who also reported muscle pain and weakness.	What is the diagnosis?	If the child does not have an infectious disease, such as rubella or measles, dermatomyositis should be considered. The diagnosis is made on the basis of clinical findings and is documented by laboratory tests, which usually provide some evidence of an immune disorder and inflammation of the muscle.
An enlarged mass was palpated in the calf of a 3-year-old child.	What kind of tumor is this?	In a young child such as this, this tumor is most likely a rhabdomyosarcoma, even though the calf is not the most common site of origin of this tumor.
A mass was palpated in the calf of a 50-year-old man.	What is the most likely diagnosis?	The most common soft tissue tumor in adults is malignant fibrous histiocytoma. Liposarcoma is the second most common tumor in this population.

Chapter 21
The Nervous System

Instruction: Match the numbered words or phrases with the most appropriate lettered item. Each lettered item can be used more than once.

- A. Developmental and/or genetic disease
- B. Circulatory disorder
- C. Infectious disease
- D. Neurodegenerative disease of unknown etiology
- E. Autoimmune disease

1. Multiple sclerosis
2. Creutzfeldt-Jakob disease
3. Tabes dorsalis
4. Alzheimer's disease
5. Parkinson's disease
6. Amyotrophic lateral sclerosis
7. Subdural hematoma
8. Stroke
9. Encephalomalacia
10. Hematocephalus
11. Meningitis
12. Tay-Sachs disease
13. Phenylketonuria
14. Down's syndrome
15. Anencephaly

Answers: 1. E, 2. C, 3. C, 4. D, 5. D, 6. D, 7. B, 8. B, 9. B, 10. B, 11. C, 12. A, 13. A, 14. A, 15. A

Instruction: Choose the one best answer.

16. Axons are cytoplasmic extensions of:
    A. Astrocytes
    B. Oligodendroglia cells
    C. Microglia cells
    D. Neurons
    E. Ependymal cells

    Answer: D

17. If a normal person has blood concentration of glucose of 100 mg/dL, the concentration in the cerebrospinal fluid will be:
    A. 0 to 10 mg/dL
    B. 50 mg/dL
    C. 100 mg/dL
    D. 200 mg/dL
    E. Unpredictable

    Answer: B

18. In myelomeningocele the protrusion of the defective spinal canal contains:
    A. Skin only
    B. Meninges only
    C. Meninges and portion of the spinal cord
    D. Meninges and vertebral bodies
    E. Meninges and displaced parts of the cerebellum

    Answer: C

19. Ruptured saccular congenital aneurysms, so-called berry aneurysms, cause hemorrhage that is best classified as:
    A. Subdural
    B. Epidural
    C. Subarachnoid
    D. Intraventricular
    E. Intracerebral

    Answer: C

20. The most common cause of stroke in the U.S. is:
    A. Arterial hypertension
    B. Intracranial hypertension
    C. Atherosclerosis
    D. Congenital berry aneurysms
    E. Arteriovenous communications in the brain

    Answer: C

21. Which of the following forms of brain injury does not cause significant macroscopic or microscopic changes in the brain?
    A. Brain concussion
    B. Brain contusion
    C. Brain laceration
    D. Coup lesion
    E. Contrecoup lesion

    Answer: A

22. St. Louis encephalitis is transmitted by:
    A. Dust inhalation
    B. Mosquito bites
    C. Tick bites
    D. Sexual contact
    E. Kissing

    Answer: C

23. Which of the following diseases can be transmitted by corneal transplantation?
    A. Huntington's disease
    B. Alzheimer's disease
    C. Creutzfeldt-Jakob disease
    D. Meningococcal meningitis
    E. Parkinson's disease

    Answer: C

24. Tabes dorsalis is characterized by:
    A. Atrophy in frontal (motor) cortex
    B. Atrophy of basal ganglia
    C. Hypertrophy of putamen
    D. Atrophy of anterior horns of the spinal cord
    E. Atrophy of the posterior columns of the spinal cord

    Answer: E

25. Multiple plaques of demyelination visible by CAT scanning are typical of:
    A. Creutzfeldt-Jakob disease
    B. Huntington's disease
    C. Viral encephalitis
    D. Multiple sclerosis
    E. Brain abscess

    Answer: D

26. Korsakoff's psychosis, which usually includes amnesia, confabulation, and general mental deterioration, is typically caused by deficiency of:
    A. Vitamin A
    B. Vitamin B_1
    C. Vitamin C
    D. Vitamin D
    E. Vitamin E

    Answer: B

27. The most prominent clinical feature of Alzheimer's disease is:
    A. Ataxia
    B. Tremor
    C. Dementia
    D. Aphasia
    E. Apraxia

    Answer: C

28. In Parkinson's disease, which part of the brain shows depigmentation?
    A. Frontal cortex
    B. Occipital cortex
    C. Cerebellum
    D. Substantia nigra
    E. Medulla oblongata

    Answer: D

29. Which of the following diseases is inherited as an autosomal dominant trait?
    A. Alzheimer's disease
    B. Tabes dorsalis
    C. Parkinson's disease
    D. Amyotrophic lateral sclerosis
    E. Huntington's disease

    Answer: E

30. Most primary malignant tumors of the brain originate from:
    A. Neurons
    B. Astrocytes
    C. Oligodendroglia cells
    D. Microglia cells
    E. Meninges

    Answer: B

31. The most common location of glioblastoma multiforme is:
    A. Cerebral hemisphere
    B. Pons
    C. Cerebellum
    D. Medulla oblongata
    E. Spinal cord

    Answer: A

32. Highly malignant tumors exclusively found in the cerebellum of children are called:
    A. Glioblastoma multiforme
    B. Medulloblastoma
    C. Ependymoma
    D. Oligodendroglioma
    E. Meningioma

    Answer: B

33. Which of the following tumors can be surgically resected with no residual consequences?
    A. Astrocytoma
    B. Oligodendroglioma
    C. Ependymoma
    D. Medulloblastoma
    E. Meningioma

    Answer: E

34. Which of the following tumors occurs only in peripheral nerves?
    A. Meningioma
    B. Oligodendroglioma
    C. Schwannoma
    D. Medulloblastoma
    E. Ependymoma

    Answer: C

Clinicopathologic Review

Chapter 21—The Nervous System

Symptoms/Findings	Question	Answer
A baby born with a small skin defect on her lower back could not move her legs.	What is the cause of her congenital paralysis?	Most likely, the skin ulcer is related to a developmental spinal cord defect that has interrupted the innervation of muscles. The exact diagnosis cannot be made without further studies, but it is likely that the baby has spina bifida.

Symptoms/Findings *(con't)*	Question *(con't)*	Answer *(con't)*
A hypertensive 60-year-old man suddenly developed an excruciating headache, collapsed, and became unconscious.	What is the cause of this man's collapse?	Most likely, he had a stroke and an intracerebral hemorrhage, which is a common complication of hypertension. Other intracranial lesions (e.g., tumors) should be considered as well.
A 65-year-old man was hospitalized with left-sided hemiparesis that developed 3 weeks after he had a massive myocardial infarct.	Is the hemiparesis related to the myocardial infarct?	Possibly. The cause of hemiparesis is most likely a cerebral infarct. The infarct could be related to an embolus originating from a thrombus overlying the infarcted myocardium of the left ventricle. However, myocardial infarction usually occurs in patients who have generalized atherosclerosis. It is possible, therefore, that the brain infarct arose from thrombotic occlusion of an atherosclerotic cerebral artery.
A 20-year-old woman had a car accident. When she was removed from the car, she could not move her legs.	Is she paralyzed for life?	Most likely, yes. Most posttraumatic paralyses occur because of complete transection of the spinal cord. Because the nerve cells cannot regenerate, the consequences of the injury are permanent.
A 30-year-old woman had a bout of flu accompanied by fever and nasal congestion. On the third day of her disease, she experienced severe headache, blurry vision, and neck rigidity.	What is the cause of these symptoms?	Most likely, this woman has developed viral meningitis. Her headache and blurred vision reflect intracranial hypertension. Stiffening of the neck is a sign of meningeal irritation. Viral meningitis is actually quite common, but it is usually mild and transitory, and often remains clinically unrecognized.
A 30-year-old woman had an episode of blurred vision, followed a month later by an episode of urinary incontinence. She recovered, but later presented complaints of tingling in her left leg.	What is the diagnosis?	In a young woman, transient symptoms of this kind could represent multiple sclerosis. Additional tests should be performed to confirm or exclude the diagnosis. MRI, electrophysiologic testing, and/or CSF analysis should be performed.

Symptoms/Findings *(con't)*	Question *(con't)*	Answer *(con't)*
The family of a 70-year-old man noticed that he had become very forgetful. He could not remember anything and was dismissed from his office job.	What is the diagnosis?	This elderly man most likely has a form of dementia. Dementia is most often a manifestation of Alzheimer's disease or cerebral atherosclerosis (multi-infarct dementia). Other, less common causes of dementia should be excluded, however.
A 55-year-old man who was becoming progressively obtunded had outbursts of bellicose behavior. He also complained that he was being persecuted by angels. One day, he killed his wife. Subsequently, he fainted and was brought to the hospital comatose. A CT scan disclosed a frontal lobe mass.	What is the diagnosis?	This patient's psychiatric symptoms and personality changes were most likely related to the mass detected by CT scan. This mass could be a brain tumor; a brain biopsy should be performed to confirm the diagnosis. Brain tumors are a well-known cause of delirium (acute confusional state), personality changes, and dementia, all of which were clinically expressed in this patient.

Chapter 22
The Eye

Instruction: Choose the one best answer.

1. The sensory innermost layer of the eye composed of rods and cones is called:
   A. Iris
   B. Cornea
   C. Sclera
   D. Retina
   E. Choroid

   Answer: D

2. Which of the following disorders has no defined underlying pathology?
   A. Glaucoma
   B. Myopia
   C. Cataract
   D. Trachoma
   E. Conjunctivitis

   Answer: B

3. Allergic conjunctivitis is typically mediated by:
   A. T lymphocytes
   B. IgA
   C. IgE
   D. IgG
   E. IgM

   Answer: C

4. Senile macular degeneration of the elderly, a common cause of blindness, is:
   A. Immune-mediated
   B. Caused by diabetes
   C. Of unknown pathogenesis
   D. Found only in myopic persons
   E. Caused by high blood pressure

   Answer: C

5. Which part of the eye is usually affected by chemical injury with exogenous caustic substances?
   A. Cornea
   B. Iris
   C. Posterior chamber
   D. Optic nerve
   E. Retina

   Answer: A

6. The most important cause of ulcerative keratitis is:
   A. CMV
   B. Herpesvirus
   C. Mumps virus
   D. Influenza virus
   E. Human papillomavirus

   Answer: B

7. Hard exudates, macular stars, and papilledema caused by arterial hypertension are best diagnosed by:
   A. Measuring the intraocular pressure
   B. Ophthalmoscopic examination of the fundus
   C. Measuring of the pupillary reflexes
   D. Measuring the vision with vision charts
   E. Biopsy of the cornea

   Answer: B

8. Which of the following is found in all patients with glaucoma?
   A. Myopia
   B. Mydriasis
   C. Hypermetropia
   D. Opacities of the lens
   E. Increased intraocular pressure

   Answer: E

9. The most important complication of untreated glaucoma is:
   A. Conjunctivitis
   B. Keratitis
   C. Iridocyclitis
   D. Retinitis
   E. Loss of eyesight

   Answer: E

10. The most common cause of cataracts in the U.S. is:
    A. Old age
    B. Trauma
    C. Endophthalmitis
    D. Trachoma
    E. Radiation

    Answer: A

11. Which of the following diseases is the most important cause of cataracts?
    A. Amyloidosis
    B. Anthracosis
    C. Diabetes mellitus
    D. Gout
    E. Hyperthyroidism

    Answer: C

12. A primary malignant tumor of the eye in a 3-month-old child is most likely a:
    A. Melanoma
    B. Basal cell carcinoma
    C. Squamous cell carcinoma
    D. Retinoblastoma
    E. Glioblastoma

    Answer: D

13. Which is the most common primary malignant intraocular tumor of adults?
    A. Meningioma
    B. Retinoblastoma
    C. Melanoma
    D. Angiosarcoma
    E. Lymphoma

    Answer: C

Clinicopathologic Review

Chapter 22—The Eye

Symptoms/Findings	Questions	Answers
A mentally retarded child had slanted eyes, a medial palpebral fold, and a speckled iris.	What is the diagnosis?	Most likely, this child has Down's syndrome, which often presents with typical eye changes. The clinical diagnosis must, however, be confirmed by karyotyping.
A man who did not wear any protective gear while sandblasting complained of eye pain. The eyes were red, and a slit lamp examination by an ophthalmologist revealed corneal scratches.	Will this eye injury have permanent consequences?	Probably not. Most corneal abrasions caused by dust or foreign material wedged between the eyelids and the surface of the eye heal spontaneously. Eye droplets with antibiotics are used to keep the eye moist and prevent infection. The eye should be kept closed to allow healing.
A 20-year-old man presented with red, swollen eyes that were extremely itchy. He reported that this itchy disease recurred in April of every year.	What is the diagnosis?	Most likely, this man has hay fever (i.e., an allergy to pollen). Hay fever presents with rhinitis, conjunctivitis, or both.
An 80-year-old woman complained of blurry vision. She did not have diabetes and was otherwise healthy.	What is the cause of her blurred vision?	Diminished visual acuity is very common in the elderly, and it may be caused by many eye diseases. The diagnosis can be made only by ophthalmoscopic examination. One should consider several possibilities, including glaucoma, cataract, or senile macular degeneration.
An infant was born with a "cat-like" whitish pupil.	What is the diagnosis?	The white material in the pupil is most likely a congenital cataract, but it could also represent a retinoblastoma. The infant should be examined by an ophthalmologist.

Chapter 23
The Ear

Instruction: Choose the one best answer.

1. Tympanic cavity is part of the:
   A. Auricle
   B. External ear
   C. Auditory meatus
   D. Middle ear
   E. Internal ear

   Answer: D

2. Earwax is secreted by:
   A. Lacrimal glands
   B. Ceruminous glands
   C. Auditory ossicles
   D. Cochlea
   E. Eustachian tube

   Answer: B

3. Malleus, incus, and stapes are located in the:
   A. Auricle
   B. Auditory canal
   C. Middle ear
   D. Inner ear
   E. Externally to the eardrum

   Answer: C

4. Otosclerosis involves all the following except:
   A. Malleus
   B. Incus
   C. Stapes
   D. Oval window
   E. Acoustic nerve

   Answer: E

5. The most typical feature of Meniere's disease is:
   A. Deafness
   B. Vertigo
   C. Strabismus
   D. Otosclerosis
   E. Acoustic hallucinations

   Answer: B

6. Conductive hearing loss may be caused by:
   A. Impacted cerumen
   B. Streptomycin
   C. Antimalarial drugs
   D. Tumor of the acoustic nerve
   E. Brain injury

   Answer: A

7. Sensory hearing loss may be a consequence of:
   A. Perforation of tympanic membrane
   B. Infection of the external auditory canal
   C. Cholesteatoma
   D. Noise trauma
   E. Laceration of the auricle

   Answer: D

8. Neural hearing loss is a feature of:
   A. Otosclerosis
   B. Cholesteatoma
   C. Otitis media
   D. Multiple sclerosis
   E. Presbycusis

   Answer: D

9. Which of the following tumors may cause vertigo?
   A. Squamous cell carcinoma of the auricle
   B. Basal cell carcinoma of the external ear
   C. Schwannoma of the VIII nerve
   D. Neurilemoma of the VII nerve
   E. Pituitary adenoma

   Answer: C

10. Sensory hearing loss of unknown etiology that affects the elderly is called:
    A. Glaucoma
    B. Otosclerosis
    C. Presbycusis
    D. Meniere's disease
    E. Vertigo

    Answer: C

Clincopathologic Review

Chapter 23—The Ear

Symptoms/Findings	Questions	Answers
A 45-year-old man woke up one morning with a loss of hearing on the right side.	What is the cause of this hearing loss?	The diagnosis cannot be made without an otologic examination. Most likely, however, the hearing loss is the result of impaction of the auditory canal with cerumen.
A 20-year-old college student was practicing for a swimming meet when she developed pain in one ear. The pain became throbbing and a fever developed.	What is the diagnosis?	Most likely, she has otitis media that is a consequence of otitis externa (swimmer's ear). An otoscopic examination of the eardrum must be performed to confirm the diagnosis.
During his annual attack of hay fever every August, a 20-year-old man also experienced itching in the ear canal.	What is the reason for the ear itch?	Most likely, he has an allergic otitis. Allergic reactions of the nose are often associated with inflammation of the eustachian tube and of the outer and middle ear.
A veteran rock star experienced loss of hearing in both ears.	What happened?	Acoustic trauma may cause sensory deafness.
A boxer who sustained a blow to the ear experienced a sudden loss of hearing.	What is the cause of his hearing loss?	Most likely, this man's deafness was caused by bleeding into the middle ear. Such an event may cause a hearing loss that is usually temporary and that lasts until the blood has been resorbed.